Recover from burnout
and get back to your best

# RISE
## AND
# SHINE

### LEANNE SPENCER

# RETHINK PRESS

First published in Great Britain 2015
by Rethink Press (www.rethinkpress.com)

Author Photo © Leanne Dixon Photography

# CONTENTS

# AUTHOR'S NOTE

My objectives in writing this book are to educate executives and their families on the dangers of burnout, to help them identify the warning signs, and to understand what they can do to recover. I am not a scientist, and I do not have any formal qualifications in medicine, psychology or biology. I've written the book based on my own personal experiences and the anecdotal experiences of others. The contents of this book are accurate to my knowledge, but where I have included the results and findings of scientific trials and studies, I have quoted the sources, and I have tried where possible to get facts and scientific statements confirmed by experts. If I have used examples of previous clients or friends, then I have asked for and obtained their written consent. In some instances, names may have been changed at the request of the person concerned but their stories are all real. It is my hope that this book will be of use to executives who think they may be suffering from burnout, and will be invaluable in helping them to recover, as well as helping people to understand more about the increasingly prevalent condition.

# INTRODUCTION

*"Through sustained focus and meditation on our patterns, habits and conditioning, we gain knowledge and understanding of our past and how we can change the patterns that aren't serving us to live more freely and fully."*

*(Yoga Sutra, III:18)*

Do you feel that your work/life balance is increasingly out of kilter? Are you already off work or on long-term sick leave with stress-related problems or anxiety or depression? Perhaps you're already suffering from burnout, so if these words resonate with you, then you need to put the brakes on now and take action.

Professional burnout is now a major problem in the City and the corporate world. According to a Health & Safety Executive Report, in the twelve months from 2013 to 2014 there were 487,000 cases of work-related stress, anxiety and depression. During the same period the total cost to the economy in terms of lost productivity was estimated at

£11.3m. In 2014 alone, 244,000 new cases of work-related stress were reported. It's not just about lost productivity; if people are out of work then they often need to be financially supported, and the oversubscribed resources of the NHS bear the strain of the costs of medication and counselling. More crucially, lost or wasted talent constitutes a huge and immoral human cost.

The City culture is spiralling out of control. We work longer and longer hours, with bonus and compensation schemes rewarding those who put in the longest day and make the greatest sacrifices. Arianna Huffington joked about the machismo amongst corporate men and women in her TED Talk in 2010; she mocked colleagues who brag about only getting four hours sleep, or who consider an 8:00am breakfast meeting to be late. There is still a lot of pressure to be the first in and last out of the office, and smartphones and the Blackberry mean that we are connected twenty-four hours a day, seven days a week in almost any part of the world. I once lay on the deck of a boat in the Mediterranean listening to the woman next to me organising a sales conference with a supplier. There are very few places to escape anymore.

The executive and their family pay the ultimate price. Professional burnout leads to uncontrolled levels of stress, anxiety and depression; jobs and careers come under threat or are lost, relationships suffer and collapse. Alarming levels of the stress hormone cortisol and adrenal fatigue lead to a highly compromised central nervous system which simply can't defend itself from illness. The risk factor for preventable disease is also much higher for people in this state; professional burnout results in low or suppressed appetite, and the body is less able to absorb the nutrients required to sustain it. Low or no levels of exercise only serve to compound the problem and leave the person feeling even more under-energised and sick. What you have left is someone who is unemployed or on sick leave; has very little self-esteem, confidence or self-worth; is struggling to find meaning in their life and their relationships; has little or no energy; eats sporadically and poorly; is over-reliant on alcohol, caffeine and nicotine, and has a dopamine addiction fed by an obsession with mobile devices, social media and email. So where do we go from here?

If you're reading this thinking, 'this is me' and starting to feel anxious and panicky, don't worry. Making the decision to read this book is a massive first step, and as you progress through the chapters, you'll read about my personal experience and what I did to turn my life around, and discover what you can do to help yourself. For ten years I worked for large corporate and financial services companies based in the City of London. In that time I sold to and managed some of the company's largest customers, and closed deals worth hundreds of thousands of pounds. All of this required time spent in the office, at a computer, and in the local wine bars networking and entertaining. After realising that my own stress levels were incredibly high, I recognised the inescapable truth that my life was out of control after several years of worsening stress, poor diet and heavy alcohol consumption. If you like, I hit my 'rock bottom'.

That was in the early part of 2012. Since then I've radically changed my life by reviewing aspects of my lifestyle that were damaging; re-igniting my passion for life and strengthening myself physically and mentally by following the steps outlined in this book; and empowering myself to want to maintain good health and happiness. I did this partly by asking for other people's help, and I would recommend that you do the same. You'll see this theme running throughout the book; there is a remarkable power at force when two people focus on a common goal with an unswerving desire to make it happen.

The framework behind my success is the methodology based on the title of this book: the Rise Method™. I adopt a principle that helps to empower people through movement; it's a feelings-based approach to personal training and recovery that centres on the client, and the key conversations that take place early in the process as well as throughout it. The core components of the approach look at balancing life-load and providing appropriate support; providing bespoke nutritional plans based on genetic testing; the inclusion of soft tissue therapies such as massage; and tailored yoga sessions to focus on quietening the mind and relaxing the body. I believe that exercise can be the most powerful mind-altering drug there is, and that the combination of empowerment and movement can alter lives in a profound way.

In this book, I'll show you the formula I use to help my clients recover from professional burnout, and go on to lead successful lives and careers. I'll also talk about how to recognise the warning signals that indicate you could be heading for burnout. The book contains case studies from people who talk candidly about their experiences and how my Rise Method™ helped them rebuild their lives. The book also includes anecdotes and quotations and each chapter is structured to cover the core principles of the framework, with useful tips from experts as well as clients, and the opportunity for self-reflection. All of this is supported with suggestions for further reading. This book is a must-read for anyone in a high-pressure environment, at any level. Whether you're just starting to see the tell-tale signs of burnout, or are already suffering its crippling effects, this book will help you to get clarity about where you currently are in life, and give you the opportunity to benefit from my proven framework for a successful recovery. The underlying message carried throughout the book is that everyone has the ability to change their lives if they have a strong desire and belief that they can.

# 1. WHAT IS BURNOUT?

*"Busy-ness is our drug of choice, numbing our minds just enough to keep us from dwelling on all that we fear we can't change. A compilation of coping mechanisms, we have become our fatigue."*

L.M. Browning, Seasons of Contemplation:
A Book of Midnight Meditations

As I established in the introduction, professional burnout is sadly not uncommon. The increasing prevalence of burnout is in large part due to aggressive and demanding aspects of the modern corporate culture that have become endemic in industries such as banking and finance, law and to a degree, amongst large accountancy and audit firms. Burnout is defined by the *Merriam-Webster Medical Dictionary* as exhaustion of physical or emotional strength or motivation usually as a result of prolonged stress or frustration. Burnout is a progressive condition which, if left unchecked and not acted upon, can result in a complete breakdown of the central nervous system. It is a very dangerous and health-span reducing condition that at best blights lives and at worst can result in loss of life. The signs and symptoms of burnout are often highly visible, but they can be easy to ignore, particularly if you're working in an aggressive corporate culture where any sign of strain might be perceived as weakness or an inability to do the job. There may also be a fear of loss of financial earnings. The symptoms of burnout are also easier to conceal if you live alone, as often the presence of a spouse, friend or family member means that you might be more likely to have a confidante, and that person will see abnormal behaviour and potentially take action.

## Measuring burnout

Social psychologists Christina Maslach and Susan Jackson developed the most widely used instrument for assessing burnout, namely, the Maslach Burnout Inventory. The Maslach Burnout Inventory defines burnout as a three-dimensional syndrome made up of exhaustion, cynicism, and inefficacy. (Maslach, 1996). In a study entitled, *The evaluation of an individual burnout intervention program; the role of inequality and social support*, burnout was recognised to be a serious threat, and specifically for employees who work with people (Van Dierendonck, 1993). It is considered to be the result of an individual's unsuccessful attempts to mediate environmental stressors (Levert, 2000). Personality traits are also related to coping mechanisms, and past experiences are relevant. Research has identified five key personality traits which can be applied when studying the effects of burnout and what types of people will be most vulnerable to it. The traits include Neuroticism, Extraversion, Openness to Experience, Agreeableness and Conscientiousness (Costa, 1987) (John, 1992).

## Classic warning signs

### Stress

The first sign that problems might be occurring is in stress levels. Feeling under pressure can be a normal part of life, and can often drive you to action and get results. When you become overwhelmed by the pressure, or your health starts to suffer, this can turn into a problem, or a stress-related condition. The NHS website defines stress as:

> 'Stress is the feeling of being under too much mental or emotional pressure.
>
> Pressure turns into stress when you feel unable to cope. People have different ways of reacting to stress, so a situation that feels stressful to one person may be motivating to someone else.'

When the body is under stress, it releases adrenaline, which causes rapid changes to the blood flow, increases your heart rate and therefore breathing, and can cause other unpleasant feelings such as clamminess, dry mouth and sweatiness. Too much adrenaline can make you feel nervous, anxious and triggers the 'fight or flight' response. The effects of stress can be managed by understanding the triggers, and by trying to remove them; by learning to relax, using exercise to manage stress levels, and being mindful of how you're feeling. The stress hormone is called cortisol, and a build-up of this can cause problems over time, so it's very important to manage your stress levels. The fires that cause burnout are always started by the spark that is stress. I'll talk more about this and a condition called adrenal fatigue later in the book.

## Anxiety

Anxiety often accompanies stress, and can be very debilitating. Like stress, anxiety is something we all experience sometimes, prior to an interview or a hospital appointment for example. It can help us to ensure we are well-prepared, and can prevent us from becoming complacent. Excessive anxiety can be very toxic however; your sleep patterns, external relationships, appetite and feeling about the larger world in general can all be adversely affected. If your anxiety levels stay high for a prolonged period, you might find it hard to deal with everyday life and feel out of control. This can lead to panic attacks, a fear of going out, and depression.

## Apathy and lack of engagement

Apathy and lack of engagement are classic signs of burnout and depression. When you're strung out and becoming increasingly run down, doing anything can seem difficult, and making the commitment to starting something, (let alone seeing it through to completion) can seem impossible. This can manifest itself in work, social life, in your personal life and in relationships. Becoming quiet and insular is not unusual, which can further exacerbate the problem.

## Cynicism

It's not unusual to become cynical and angry when you're feeling burned out. A lot of the joy can disappear from life and you fail to see the humour in anything. This is hardly surprising. Often this can be misinterpreted as aggression, and relationships often suffer as a result.

## Insomnia or poor sleep

Insomnia and broken sleep can be a real and present danger. In my experience, it can be very hard to change anything if you're sleep-starved and walking around like a zombie during the day or are wired up to the eyeballs with caffeine and sugar. Sadly, people suffering from burnout and extreme stress frequently use sugar and caffeine as props to get them through the day. Sugar and caffeine can be very addictive, psychologically and physically, and a diet heavy on both can have health repercussions, of which diabetes, metabolic diseases and malnutrition are just a few.

## Erratic eating

I find that healthy eating is one of the first things to go awry when the early signs of burnout show themselves. A busy and demanding working life (and home life) often means that fitting in regular meals can be difficult. Cortisol, the stress hormone, has the effect of suppressing appetite, so that you don't feel hungry. Combine this with feelings of extreme tiredness and apathy, and it's easy to see how food of any kind can drop down the list of priorities. Cortisol also affects blood sugar levels; fat, carbohydrate and protein absorption; the immune system responses; blood pressure; heart rate variation, and anti-inflammatory actions. If cortisol levels are out of balance, the consequences can be severe. Cortisol is secreted by the adrenal glands which play an important function in good health – more on that in the next section.

## Adrenal Fatigue

The adrenal glands are two small glands which sit above the kidneys and are each about the same size as a large grape. They can be found beneath your back ribs towards the spine. The adrenal glands secrete cortisol, but over time as stress levels rise unchecked, the glands become fatigued and cease to function properly. This has a profound effect on every organ in the body, and the immune system becomes severely compromised. The person becomes very vulnerable to sickness and disease. At its worst, adrenal fatigue can leave you utterly unable to get out of bed; this is a classic symptom of burnout.

## Low energy/exhaustion

Extreme tiredness, stress, and a heavy workload take their toll on energy levels, compounded by all the other factors such as work, travel, family demands and so on. Exhaustion manifests itself when the adrenal glands are fatigued and cannot carry on their everyday job, and your body starts to shut down. Poor nutritional choices and excessive caffeine can also have an influence on energy levels.

## Excessive worrying, self-criticism

Once you start to become burned out or extremely stressed, small things that ordinarily would be manageable can appear much bigger. You lose your sense of perspective, can become more cynical and pessimistic, and can also develop a tendency to catastrophise about events. Often this will come across as very unlike you and people may remark upon it.

## Inefficacy

Efficacy is defined in *Wikipedia* as, 'The capacity for beneficial change'. When you're under extreme stress, it's easy to start thinking you're no good at anything, or likely to fail. Chances are you might have started to struggle at things that ordinarily you would excel at or find easy. Your stressed-out brain, tired, undernourished and thriving on adrenaline, will make mistakes more readily and be less likely to think clearly and make sensible, rational decisions.

## Forgetfulness and impaired concentration

The brain depends on glucose to operate normally. It gets glucose from the foods you eat, which is why you struggle to think clearly when you're hungry. The key role of glucose in the body is fuel for energy, and although it only accounts for about 2% of our body weight, the brain requires about 20% of our recommended daily calorie intake to keep functioning optimally. (Incidentally, this is about twice as much energy as that required by any other organ). This is because the brain is rich in neurons, or nerve cells, and these cells expend energy to create specialised enzymes and proteins in order to function. Stress, or more specifically an excess of cortisol, can also interfere with your ability to encode memories. Cortisol is a common biomarker for stress, and belongs to a class of stress hormones called glucocorticoids. Under normal circumstances, the hippocampus, a part of the brain that deals with short and long term memory among other important functions, regulates the production of cortisol through negative feedback because it has many receptors that are sensitive to these stress hormones. However, an excess of cortisol can impair the ability of the hippocampus to both encode and recall memories. These stress hormones are also hindering the hippocampus from receiving enough energy by diverting glucose levels to surrounding muscles.

**Anger and irritability**

Anger can be caused by many things, often circumstantial, such as being passed up for promotion, relationship problems, or when we perceive our self-esteem, authority or reputation is being questioned. A certain degree of irritability or anger is fairly normal, uncontrolled anger is not. Often this stems from a perceived loss of control, both internal and external. When you're living on your nerves, it's easy to get frustrated when things aren't going to plan, or you don't feel you have time to do anything, least of all properly. There's often a lot more going on behind anger though, and usually it's being driven by fear and anxiety. Anger can be a symptom of anxiety and also a cause; if you suffer from anger management issues, you're probably also caught up in a lot of anxiety about that. Loss of temper, or extreme bursts of anger, can often lead people into trouble with the law or result in actual harm, so this is a very dangerous symptom of burnout.

## Anhedonia

Anhedonia is defined by the *Mirriam-Webster Medical Dictionary* as being, 'a psychological condition characterised by an inability to experience pleasure in acts which normally produce it.' Anhedonia is also a symptom of major depression disorder, and it is believed to be caused by the brain closing down its pleasure circuits. It can be exacerbated by adrenal fatigue, and some of the other signs and symptoms of burnout. Very often you'll hear people under extreme stress report that they struggle to get pleasure from anything, even activities that they have loved in the past.

## Numbness of feeling

Often linked to anhedonia, when you're burned out you can feel numb to your feelings and emotions. You might also struggle to relate or empathise with the significant emotional events that occur to others, towards which you might ordinarily be sympathetic.

## Isolation & Detachment

As I will explore later in the book, burnout can occur more frequently in people who live alone, predominantly because the symptoms can go unchecked for longer, and because of the absence of a partner, spouse or flatmate to offload onto or relax with after work. Lack of energy can contribute to a reluctance to socialise, and you might also feel unable to connect with others due to your feelings of stress, anxiety and exhaustion. If you are self-medicating with large amounts of alcohol, this might also lead to secretive and unsocial behaviours.

# Personality, Temperament & Childhood Origins

## Personality

In my experience and in the course of researching this book, I've found a number of commonalities amongst the personality types. There are things that happen to us in childhood that mould and influence our thoughts, behaviours, actions and decisions well into adulthood. This can work very positively for us but can also be at the root of some very negative and damaging behaviour. In her excellent book *Fried*, Joan Borysenko PhD writes:

*"My childhood experiences, in combination with in-born temperament and external environment, put me at very high risk of burnout... I'm hardwired to overachieve, search for perfection, and crash and burn repeatedly."*

Research shows that there are commonalities amongst personality traits that are markers for burnout; when people with these personality traits are put into a stressful environment, they are more likely than others to suffer from emotional exhaustion or burnout.

A psychologist whom I met a number of years ago described burnout as the result of, 'being too strong for too long'. Often this 'strength' has been in place for a long time, and in the end it can prove to be our greatest strength and our greatest weakness. This was certainly the case for me; if I hadn't been so high-functioning then I would have perhaps planned my exit from my career much sooner than I did and spared myself some difficult times.

## Key personality traits

### Know when to let go!

If prolonged and chronic stress is present, there is a very good chance that the individual has allowed the stressor to remain present. I think this is particularly true when applied to both relationships (professional and personal) and careers. All too often I see my clients staying in jobs that are causing them misery, placing extreme and intolerable amounts of stress upon them and making them sick. It's not at all uncommon for a client to relay a story about how they were on their way to a meeting or to the office only to stop still in the street, unable to continue or unable to remember where they were going. Quite often, that person will remain in their job for many weeks, months or even years after the signs of burnout have appeared, because it's very hard to know when to let go. I probably spent three or four years working in a stressful and high-pressure environment, with which I didn't fit or belong, purely because I didn't know how to let go, and for a long while, wrongly believed that I couldn't.

## Stuck in a velvet rut

The velvet rut was a term used by a friend of mine many years ago and I think it's a wonderfully descriptive metaphor. On the face of it, a person suffering from burnout might appear to have a very nice life. They probably have a senior position in a company or are running a successful business, and have a comfortable, spacious home in a safe area with a car, a good social life, the ability to afford luxurious holidays and to eat at good restaurants. It's also feasible that they have children, and those children go to expensive schools. Despite this, that person might well find themselves trapped in the velvet rut. It's a rut, because it's difficult to get out of, and it's taking you relentlessly forwards. There isn't much lateral movement, and when you do try and change direction, you typically don't get anywhere. The cushion is the burnout will have also suffered from some form of trauma in childhood. It might be a bereavement, mental or physical abuse, bullying or feeling trapped in an environment such as a boarding school where you were pushed too hard. The feelings of despair and helplessness that result from trauma in childhood become hardwired into your nervous system as an adult. Take a moment to consider your own childhood and past, and you will probably be able to identify one major event that stands out to you. Consider now how your behaviour later in life might be affected by this event, and you may well have just identified the first sparks that led to burnout. Contrary to the cliché that time heals, in the case of childhood trauma, it's probably fairer to say that time passes, but it does not heal. Instead it provides you with the opportunity to get really good at masking and concealing. Swiss psychoanalyst Alice Miller says:

'The truth about our childhood is stored up in our bodies, and lives in the depths of our souls. Our intellect can be deceived, our feelings can be numbed and manipulated, our perceptions can be shamed and confused, or our bodies tricked with medication. But our soul never forgets. And because we are one, one whole soul in one body, some day, our body will present its bill.'

## Adverse Childhood Experiences study

There is a major research project called the Adverse Childhood Experiences (ACE) study that has explored the ways in which childhood experiences have affected health later in life. The study is being managed principally by Robert F. Anda MD, MS and Vincent J. Felitti, MD and is a collaboration between the Centres for Disease Control and Prevention in Atlanta and the Kaiser Permanente. Between 1995 and 1997, just over 17,000 patients voluntarily participated in the study which involved routine screening to assess the long term health outcomes of patients who had experienced childhood neglect or abuse. The findings of the study clearly identify a link between chronic stress and poor health outcomes later in life. To formulate the ACE score, both Felitti and Anda worked with the participants to identify eight categories of adverse experience. The three abuse categories were emotional, physical and sexual. The five categories of household dysfunction included substance abuse, a household member detained in prison, a household member suffering from depression or mental illness, the death of a biological parent, or domestic abuse targeted at the mother. One point was given to each adverse experience, and if none of the experiences were relevant, no points were allocated. The average age of the participants was in their late fifties, so Felitti and Anda then correlated the scores against the health outcomes of each participant at the time of the study. What they discovered was fascinating; the ACE scores were a strong indicator of health outcomes in adulthood. In other words, the higher the score, the greater likelihood of poor health and behavioural problems in adulthood. The developing architecture of their brains was altered by the

8. **Obvious behavioural changes** – colleagues, friends and family can no longer ignore the changes that have occurred in you

9. **Depersonalisation** – you lose track of your personal needs and 'lose yourself', performing mechanical functions only and viewing life only in the present time

10. **Inner emptiness** – possibly manifesting itself in damaging behaviours such as overeating, undereating, casual sex, alcohol or drugs

11. **Depression** – you are exhausted, and can see little or no meaning in life

12. **Burnout syndrome** – this is a physical and mental collapse which requires immediate medical attention.

## Stress and burnout are not the same

### Stress

I've already established that some levels of stress are normal, necessary and can act as a safety net, ensuring we don't get complacent. When everyday stress becomes chronic stress, this is where the problems start. For the executive, low levels of stress ensure that your deadlines are met, presentations are prepared for and you stay focused on your role and responsibilities. This type of stress is often linked to a specific event, such as a project, deal or situation, and usually, once the project or deal is concluded, the stress dissipates and you recover. Research done in 2009 by Professor Ayala Malach-Pines of Ben-Gurion University in Israel found that if executives feel that their work is valuable and meaningful, then they are less likely to burnout. She says:

'The root cause of burnout lies in people's need to believe that their lives are meaningful, that the things they do are useful and important. For many people, the driving force behind their work is not merely monetary but the belief that they can have an impact, and it is this idea that spurs them on.' She goes on to add that, '...it is possible to be very stressed but not burned out if you feel your work is worthwhile and you are achieving the desired goals.'

Perhaps we should be focusing on encouraging executives to achieve a balance in their lives, and reduce the unswerving focus on short-term goals and monetary benefits rather than running people down like batteries. More on this in the next chapter.

**Burnout**

When the stressors become prolonged and continual, the risks of burning out become much greater. Where stress might be characterised by over-engagement, burnout becomes characterised by disengagement. Where stress produces a sense of urgency and hyperactivity, burnout produces feelings of helplessness and hopelessness. Stress causes a loss of energy, whereas burnout causes loss of motivation, ideals and hope. With stress, the primary damage is physical, and with burnout the primary damage is emotional. If you're burned out, you will continue to feel stressed even after the stressors have gone or lessened. You have also lost your sense of self-efficacy and can no longer see the value in what you do. In some cases it results in a total breakdown of the central nervous system, which requires medical intervention and several months or even years to fully recover.

## Diagnosis

The symptoms of burnout are often similar to that of depression. In a study by Bianchi, R., Boffy, C., Hingray, C., Truchot, D., & Laurent, E. (2013). *Comparative symptomatology of burnout and depression*: *Journal of Health Psychology, 18(6), 782-787,* there were no observable differences between clinically depressed workers and workers suffering from burnout. Diagnosis is often made by the GP; all of the people I interviewed for this book had visited their GP in the first instance (with mixed results). Commonly, the visit to the GP has been deferred until too late, and any assistance the GP might have been able to offer is too little, too late. I personally waited until the red flags were impossible to ignore before taking action, and I suspect I'm not alone in that. Sometimes anti-depressants are prescribed, along with sleeping pills or anxiety medications.

One of my case studies, Sarah, fought the suggestion by her GP that she try anti-depressants, only to find that they helped her enormously once she tried them. I believe there is a place for medication, but every individual case is different, and ultimately the executive has to decide for themself whether they think it will help them. Here's Sarah's story.

## CASE STUDY: Sarah R

Sarah is a senior lawyer working in the public sector, and is very passionate about her vocation (and is clearly also very good at it). She lives and works in London with her husband and two boys, and has the support of her friends and family. I have asked Sarah to share her experience because, whilst she hasn't suffered from burnout, her story helps to illustrate the difference between stress and burnout, and reveal the warning signs. When Sarah came to us looking for help, she was working incredibly long hours both in the office and at home, and frequently skipped meals. Her sleep patterns were erratic, and sometimes she might only get two or three hours of sleep a night. When we met, I found her to be a very honest and warm person, clearly very intelligent, but also scared and anxious. This is her experience in her own words.

I have suffered from high levels of work-related stress/ low level depression for some twelve years and I find my wellness to be cyclical. I am fine, all is well, I hit a sustained difficult period at work, my health declines, I become unwell, I battle my way through it (both the work and its impact) and I recover. And then it happens all over again.

The need to control (even more than usual!) is the first signal; I obsess over less important or less time-sensitive activities rather than tackling the critical tasks. Then comes the disruption to my sleeping. I am tired but I don't allow myself to go to bed because then the morning and the return to work comes sooner. Needless to say, the exhaustion comes next. Couple that with more erratic eating – caused by the unrelenting hours at my desk and the sleep deprived need for carbs and sugar – and, hey presto, I find myself teetering on the emotional edge.

I have given some significant thought as to whether it is 'me' or 'my job' that means I find myself in a pretty near constant cycle of wellness-stress-decline-recovery-repeat and I am still unable to come to a conclusion. I am the eldest of three girls; we are all high achievers but my parents are very much of a nurturing and supporting nature and are not at all ambitious or pushy when it comes to the way in which we live our lives. Performing to the very best of my ability is important to me. I am harder on myself than anyone else ever is. These are things which make me think it is 'me' and a number of people close to me agree; it is often said that I would have the local supermarket totally re-organised by the end of week one if I were to go back to my check-out girl years. But the career I have chosen doesn't help. I believe so very passionately in what I do and my level of commitment to my work and the people I manage together with the traits which make 'me' mean I have a complex relationship with my mental health.

Several years ago I reached a place where, despite fighting the suggestion for some considerable time, I began taking anti-depressants. My GP had been our family doctor for more than fifteen years when I first went to him complaining of a near perpetual exhaustion coupled with an inability to get a decent night's sleep. We talked several times. He diagnosed depression caused by work-related stress. I disagreed. He suggested anti-depressants. I resisted. To prove his point he prescribed a short course of sleeping tablets whilst advising me that I might feel worse. He was right. He nudged me along slowly, eventually saying, 'if you had a broken arm, would you let me set it?' to which of course the answer was yes. 'If you had a cut on your leg, would you let me bandage it?' I said yes again. 'So why won't you let me fix these broken synapses in your brain?' He had a point. I took the prescription. I started taking the tablets and they were remarkable – within just a few days I felt like me again. There is no doubt that medication worked for me – my body responded quickly and remarkably well to the SSRI (Selective Serotonin Reuptake Inhibitors, a popular type of anti-depressant commonly prescribed by the medical community) that I was prescribed but I have never felt the need/desire to take another course. People talk about the 'cloud lifting' and it very much did and I will always be grateful to a wonderful and caring GP who carefully and gently brought me through a difficult time.

I have never told my employer about my difficulties and I can't explain why. I work in the civil service whose commitment to taking care of its staff is well documented and yet I don't feel comfortable in discussing my lack of well-being. And it is perhaps worth me saying that it is not my work which suffers during these periods. I continue to work long hours, I continue to produce high quality work against difficult deadlines, I continue to manage and support my team with my usual patience and good humour. Very few people would know that I am struggling. But it is my family that suffers. My husband, parents and sisters are well attuned to the signs of a decline in my health and are quick to try to help – the difficulty is that it is only me who can bring me through these periods and it often takes a long while for me to be able to take the necessary steps to set me on the road to recovery.

In a later period, I found myself once again in a place where I sought assistance from my GP, this time in London. My experience was again positive but definitely lacked the level of personal care which I had been lucky enough to experience previously. I explained that I did not want to take medication unless her advice was unequiv-ocal that it was the right thing for me and instead she prescribed a course of Cognitive Behavioural Therapy (CBT). (Author's note: CBT is a form of psychotherapy that teaches you to solve your problems by changing the way you think and behave). I had six sessions and, whilst I think it helped me in getting through at the time, I do not think that the therapy has had any lasting effect. I have also, periodically, seen a reflexologist. I cannot say whether I get any medical benefit from it but the calm that lying down quietly brings certainly relieves the strain for the occasional hour.

The on/off battle I have had with high levels of stress/low level depression over twelve years had taken its toll on my physical health – the combination of poor sleeping habits, poor eating habits and not exercising meant that I was unfit and carrying too much weight. But that same battle is what led me, only six months ago, to the website of a personal trainer. I was just about to take on a new role at work (not a promotion but a substantially different and significantly more responsible role) and I knew that I needed to be fitter, stronger and better able to cope with the strains that I knew would be heading my way. And being brave enough to take myself out of my comfort zone and to book a course of personal training sessions is one of the best decisions of my life.

The real change has come with exercise. Whether it is the impact of taking some time out of my otherwise hectic life; the fact that there are no decisions to be made during those hours; the effect of being outside in the fresh air; the endorphin rush; the sense of achievement; the improved sleep pattern; the resultant desire to eat well – all of those things together mean that I feel calmer and am better able to cope with the stress caused by my job than I have ever been able to previously.

The key to staying well is to achieve and maintain balance. That isn't easy to do given our lifestyles so we must recognise when we start to feel the balance getting out of kilter and take early steps to restore it. If we can't recognise it in ourselves, we must listen to the people who love us when they try to tell us that they are worried about us.

Despite being very aware of my own physical and mental health and being knowledgeable about all the medical advice, I still struggle to bring a halt to this constant cycle of wellness-stress-decline-recovery-repeat. But I do think, through exercising, that I might finally have found the key to more constant wellbeing.

# 2. CORPORATE LANDSCAPE

## A Day in the Life of an Executive

*'Greed, for lack of a better word, is good. Greed is right. Greed works. Greed clarifies, cuts through, and captures, the essence of the evolutionary spirit. Greed, in all of its forms; greed for life, for money, for love, knowledge, has marked the upward surge of mankind and greed, you mark my words, will not only save Teldar Paper, but that other malfunctioning corporation called the U.S.A.'*

*Gordon Gekko, (Wall Street)*

So we've all probably watched the film *Wall Street* or at least heard about its main protagonist, the ruthless Gordon Gekko. The film *Wolf of Wall Street* also did little to improve the image of your average executive (working in the financial markets). Executives in these films are portrayed as ruthless, self-obsessed, hedonistic, greedy and self-serving. At the time of writing, one of the executives from the real-life *Wolf of Wall Street* story, a fifty-two-year old man named William 'Preston' King, was found sleeping on a park bench in Greenwich Village, New York. According to news reports, his addictions to drugs and alcohol got the better of him and he's now unemployed and homeless. King was a very successful broker for firms like Merrill Lynch, and was an associate of the so-called Wolf of Wall Street, Jordan Belfont. When Belfont heard the news reports, he said this:

'There was so much partying back then. That journey into coke is just so destructive, makes you paranoid. I thought there were aliens coming in my window. I went crazy, was completely out of touch with reality before I got sober.'

Whilst these tales of depravity and excess are not uncommon, the reality is perhaps a little different. We will all either know or work with executives who fit that bill, but a lot are decent, hardworking and honest people who find themselves in jobs that don't fulfil their basic needs and don't allow them any opportunity to balance their lifestyles in a healthy and sustainable way.

## Competitive presenteeism

Can you think of a scenario in your office where someone has turned up for work quite clearly ill? They might be sneezing, clutching their pounding head whilst stirring in an Alka Seltzer, or even suffering from the early effects of exhaustion because of sleep problems? If they're evidently very sick, you might wonder why they came into the office instead of staying at home in bed. I can recall many times when that happened and I'd hear grandiose remarks such as 'I can't afford to stay in bed' or 'I've got too much to do' or 'I'm not staying at home in bed when I've got X, Y or Z to do here'. Arianna Huffington takes this even further in her TED Talk of December 2010:

'There is now a kind of sleep deprivation one-upmanship. Especially here in Washington, if you try and make a breakfast date, and you say, 'How about eight o'clock?' they're likely to tell you, 'eight o'clock is too late for me, but that's okay, I can get a game of tennis in and do a few conference calls and meet you at eight.' And they think that means that they are so incredibly busy and productive, but the truth is they're not, because we, at the moment, have had brilliant leaders in business, in finance, in politics, making terrible decisions. So a high I.Q. does not mean that you're a good leader, because the essence of leadership is being able to see the iceberg before it hits the Titanic. And we've had far too many icebergs hitting our Titanics.'

Competitive presenteeism is now endemic in the corporate world. It's a game of 'how sick can you be and still come into the office', or 'who can survive on the least amount of sleep'. I've experienced it first hand in all of the offices I've worked in, and I'm willing to bet you have too. And the stark fact is that quite often, in some environments, they will be the people recognised as the hardest workers, the ones who put the hours in and are therefore most committed. I hear all the time of my clients unable to say no to employers when asked to work late because of the fear of consequences, and because they know that if they don't say yes, they will lose out on future opportunities or be deemed to be disinterested and uncommitted. There's something interesting going on though, because the UK also has a problem with sick leave, so perhaps this competitive presenteeism is false economy. In 2013, big-four audit firm, PwC, conducted research that found UK workers have an average of 9.1 sick days each year, nearly double the amount workers in the US take (4.9 days) and four times more than Asia-Pacific (2.2 days). In total, sick leave was estimated to have cost UK employers about £29 billion a year in lost productivity. So whilst we do have some members of the workforce thriving on competitive presenteeism, we also have a lot of other workers too sick to come to the office. Could the two be linked? And are we pushing our executives too hard, without providing them with a culture and the tools to ensure they have a healthy balance in their lives?

## High Profile Examples

Let's look at some recent examples of high profile executives who suffered from burnout.

Antonio Horta-Osorio is the current Chief Executive of Lloyds Banking Group. He took up his post in March 2011, at a time when the bank was in a dire state; in 2008, the credit crunch that precipitated the largest financial crisis since 1929 had affected Lloyds badly and the UK government had to intervene, becoming its largest shareholder in the process.

Antonio Horta-Osorio is from Portugal, and was at the helm of the UK division of Spanish Bank Santander before he was headhunted for the Lloyds job. In his interviews he describes coming from a competitive family, and lists his interests as swimming with sharks. (This in itself might give you a clue about how hard the man drives himself in his professional life). Just over six months after his appointment however, Horta-Osorio announced he was taking a medical leave for exhaustion. He describes the issues in an interview in the *Guardian* in December 2011, shortly after his return to work:

'By the beginning of September I was beginning to have problems sleeping. I would go to bed exhausted but could not get to sleep. I could not switch off. I had never had this problem before. I was ending up with just two or three hours' sleep every night.'

Horta-Osorio eventually checked in to the Priory in West London for a five-week stay, before leaving the clinic and telling the Chairman of Lloyds that he wanted to return to work.

Interestingly, no-one in the bank used the word stress in any of the public conversations or statements that were released during the time of the medical leave. Neither does Horta-Osorio use the word stress; he describes his condition as exhaustion or insomnia. Perhaps it was felt that insomnia didn't conjure up the same connotations as stress in terms of resilience. After all, the board of directors at Lloyds would not want to admit to the stock market or their largest shareholder, (the UK Financial Investments Ltd, responsible for managing the government's shareholding in Lloyds), that their CEO was struggling with his responsibilities. Horta-Osorio was reinstated in January 2012. That followed an independent medical assessment prepared for the board and individual interviews with Horta-Osorio by each of the other sixteen directors. There were questions raised in the City about his ability to do his job as effectively, but time has gone on to prove that he has been able to manage his role and responsibilities in such a way that he hasn't needed to take further medical leave. Asked to summarise his thoughts on what might have led to his condition he said:

'With the benefit of hindsight I overdid it. I focused too much on too many details.' He adds, 'The message to people working in the City or anywhere else where they are under extreme pressure and suffering, with the benefit of hindsight, is to seek professional help immediately.' (taken from an interview with the *Guardian* newspaper, December 2011)

Hector Sants led the FSA from 2007 to 2012 before stepping down to join Barclays in a role created especially for him in compliance and government and regulatory relations. Just one month after beginning work, he left, citing 'exhaustion and stress'.

In a statement, Barclays said: 'Hector Sants has been on sick leave since the beginning of October, suffering from stress and exhaustion. He has concluded that he will not be able to return to work in the near term. Consequently he has decided to resign from Barclays and not return from sick leave.'

Not much was made of Sants' resignation, and unsurprisingly Barclays were reluctant to discuss the circumstances around his departure.

Sam Smith is a corporate broker working in London. She is widely regarded in the City, and at the age of forty-one has already achieved an enormous amount, including a management buyout of the firm JM Finn where she worked in 2007. JM Finn became FinnCap, of which Smith owns 16% (the firm is 95% owned by its staff). Smith has built a business that advises more than 100 of the UK's fastest-growing businesses, but in order to achieve this she found herself frequently working fourteen-hour days, including lunches and dinners with clients. After a holiday to South Africa, she and her fourteen-month-old daughter contracted a parasitic infection which left them very sick and, in the case of her daughter, unable to sleep properly for months. Eventually, Smith collapsed with exhaustion, and had to take two weeks off to recover, most of which she says she spent sleeping. She says, 'You can see why tiredness is a form of torture.'

Having made a full recovery, Smith is now trying to adapt the culture she works in. She says of the City, 'It's not known for its team spirit. It's still an alpha place to do business but I don't think it has to be like that. You don't have to be a ball-breaker and I don't believe in all that macho stuff.' (taken from an interview with the *Standard* newspaper, July 2011). She now says she's 'found a good balance', and this includes making herself do something every year that pushes her out of her comfort zone, to try and progress herself and keep herself motivated.

Jeff Kindler resigned from his position as Chief Executive of Pfizer in December 2010 stating he needed to recharge his batteries. He provided this statement to the press at the time:

'The combination of meeting the requirements of our stakeholders around the world and the 24/7 nature of my responsibilities, has made this period extremely demanding on me personally.'

In 2011, the Chief Executive of the UK property services group Connaught, Mark Tincknell, resigned shortly before the company collapsed. Connaught issued a statement saying Tincknell 'needed to recover from recent health issues.'

Masataka Shimizu, the president of the Tokyo Electric Power company (TEPCO), left in a controversial period for his company, citing 'a personal matter… brought on by overwork and lack of sleep.'

Joseph Lombardi was the chief financial officer of the bookstore Barnes & Noble in the US until 2011 when he abruptly resigned. 'I think he's exhausted and ready for a new challenge,' said a colleague. Whilst it's difficult to find any concrete statements about the reason behind his departure, it seems the general assumption was that he was exhausted, having fought a very public battle with a major stakeholder and been at the helm of a company that was undergoing major industry changes.

One thinks of Huffington's words about icebergs and Titanics, and wonders if there was less stigma around stress and mental health, an improved culture of work/life balance, and less competitive presenteeism and machismo, then perhaps there would be more vigilance and fewer collisions.

## All about the dopamine

If money makes the world go round, then it's dopamine that draws it to the City. Dopamine is a neurotransmitter that helps to control the brain's reward and pleasure centres, and is also a precursor of adrenaline. It's what drives a lot of us to repeat our behaviours, both good and bad. Dopamine is what we experience when we complete a large task (for example

I had a huge rush of dopamine every time I completed a section of this book and an enormous surge once it was ready for publishing). It's also the good feeling we get when someone shows interest in us romantically or when we get good news. Many of us feel that same hit of pleasure when we get a message on our mobile phones. Some even go to the extreme of repeatedly hitting the refresh button despite knowing that any new messages will be automatically delivered with an accompanying beep or buzzing sound. Believe it or not, there is even a phobia to describe the fear of losing or being without your mobile phone: nomophobia, short for 'no mobile phone phobia'. Even if you think this isn't you, you probably know someone who has nomophobia. And consider this; when did you last use a physical map, memorise a phone number or refer to a paper calendar?

Dopamine is highly addictive, so once we've felt a rush of dopamine, it's in our nature to want to recreate that feeling again and again. This is the problem with the way the banking and corporate structure is currently set up; it's configured to reward risk-taking for large capital gains, with little sense of responsibility or personal consequences. Simon Sinek, in his brilliant book *Leaders Eat Last*, describes the effects of dopamine on our brains:

'As helpful as (dopamine) is, we can also form neural connections that do not help us survive – in fact, they can actually do the complete opposite. The behaviours we reinforce can actually do us harm. Cocaine, nicotine, alcohol and gambling all release dopamine. And the feelings can be intoxicating. The chemical effects notwithstanding, the addictions we have to these things (and lots of other things that feel good) are all basically dopamine addictions. The only variation is the behaviour that is reinforced that gives us the next hit of dopamine.'

## Reward Culture Gone Mad

Recently, there have been many high-profile cases of executives who have lost control, perhaps allowing their dopamine addiction to cloud their judgement to such as extent that they have taken enormous risks with their employer's funds, resulting in exile or even prison time. Here are some recent examples:

Jérome Kerviel almost brought French investment bank Société Générale to its knees in 2008 when he was convicted of breach of trust, forgery and unauthorised use of the bank's computers and sentenced to prison for five years. He was accused of 'rogue trading', and of generating record losses of €4.9 billion to his employer. Société Générale claim he was working alone, and turned renegade, but in his book *Downward Spiral: Memoirs of a Trader*, Kerviel claims that his superiors were well aware of what he was doing and that in fact his behaviour was widespread at the bank. In various news sources, colleagues and acquaintances back up these claims, and perhaps surprisingly, Kerviel did not personally profit from his rogue trading. Whilst there was clearly wrongdoing on the part of Kerviel, we might never know how much of that was encouraged by bosses who turned a blind eye whilst big profits were being recorded, and how much of it was a trader acting on his own dopamine-fuelled greed. Many feel that Kerviel was made a scapegoat for the wider and systemic failings of the banking system; you will have to draw your own conclusions on that. In the end he was released on appeal after serving 110 days of his sentence, which equates to one day for every €50 million he lost on behalf of the bank.

Nicknamed the 'Gorilla' on Wall Street for his competitiveness, Richard (Dick) Fuld was the last Chairman and CEO of the long-standing Wall Street investment bank Lehman Brothers, which shocked the financial world when it announced it was filing for chapter 11 bankruptcy protection on the 15th September 2008. (You might recall the infamous images of stunned Lehman Brothers staff carrying their desk contents across Canary Wharf in cardboard boxes after hearing that the bank had collapsed). The demise of the Lehman Brothers Holdings, which was founded in 1850 by Henry Lehman, the son of a Jewish cattle merchant, has been largely attributed to Dick Fuld and his tyrannical, egotistical and megalomaniac style of management. In his 2009 book *A Colossal Failure of Common Sense*, Larry McDonald described Fuld as 'belligerent and unrepentant', and as

'The man in the ivory tower'. McDonald (a senior Lehman Brothers trader in the years leading up to the crash,) also writes that Fuld's 'smouldering envy' of Goldman Sachs and other Wall Street rivals led him to ignore warnings from Lehman executives about the impending crash. McDonald reported that Fuld exploded in a meeting of senior executives who were trying to work out the scale of the problem shouting 'I've had enough! Enough of the f**king losses! Enough!' It is reported that Fuld didn't understand the complex products that the bank was trading, such as Credit Default Swaps (CDS), Collaterised Loan Obligations (CLO), Residential Mortgage Backed Securities (RMBS) and Commercial Mortgage Backed Securities (CMBS). It is suggested by Larry McDonald in his book that Fuld wasn't interested in the details of the products but only in the bottom line, and once he realised the balance sheet was full of toxic junk, impossible to offload, he reverted to type and refused to accept that there was a problem. He still to this day claims to be baffled as to why Lehman was allowed to fail. It has been argued that his actions were and still are driven by ego, arrogance, vanity, disillusionment and greed. Lehman collapsed leaving 25,000 people without jobs and a staggering $613bn in bank debt and $155bm in bond debt.

Banks in general have been held to account recently with some record-breaking fines being levied against the likes of Barclays (£500m for currency fixing); JP Morgan (fined £572m for the London Whale scandal); and HSBC (£1.2bn for money laundering). In 2014, six banks were collectively fined a staggering £2.1bn for manipulating the foreign exchange markets. The general consensus is there needs to be firmer action taken against these huge banks, and more responsibility needs to be shown, starting from the top. In 2013, the Parliamentary Commission on Banking Standards reported, 'too many bankers, especially at the most senior levels, have operated in an environment of diminished responsibility.'

## Striking the balance: Paul Pester

I recently had the privilege of hearing Paul Pester speak at a workshop. He was invited to talk about how he steered the high street bank TSB through the significant changes it underwent as it moved from being part of Lloyds Banking Group to its new owner, Sabadell Bank. He is a banker with a first class honours in physics, and previously worked for McKinsey, Virgin Money and Santander, before taking up the role of TSB's Chief Executive at a relatively young age. Pester is generally considered to be a new breed of banker, who welcomes transparency and is less macho about his own working practices and what he expects of his staff. During the sale process, Paul divided his time between investment banks, meetings involving key advisors, shareholder meetings and internal meetings. He actually put up a PowerPoint slide of his diary to show us, and it was more or less booked up with meetings, with a few gaps for travel time. The first meeting started at 7.30am and the last sometimes finished after 9pm. He did however have a few gaps, shaded in different colours from the rest of the diary. These gaps were for swimming sessions (he is a skilled swimmer, and has been since childhood). Keeping these swim sessions in whenever he could, he told us, helped him to maintain his good health and stay focused, resilient and sharp during what was a very busy and stressful period. As a general rule he tries to swim in London on a Thursday evening and also trains on a Saturday near his family home in Norfolk. He also does triathlons, cycles and runs as a way of keeping himself mentally and physically fit and healthy.

During his talk, Pester gave us an insight into how he manages his working life, and what enabled him to stay level headed and healthy during the sale of TSB. He called it his survival plan, which he described in three separate areas:

**Effectiveness** – setting priorities, having a shortlist of actions and focusing only on what he personally had to do. He quoted his mentor, who said write an A list, a B list and a C list and then review them. Rip up the C list, rip up the B list and concentrate only on the A list. In other words, if someone else can do it then let them.

**Efficiency** – build and cultivate a strong team around you. Encourage pyramid training amongst executives. Ensure all documents have a standardised front page; this means all documents have to be summarised or presented in a standard format ensuring the reader can quickly grasp the contents and determine whether they need to take action. This saves a lot of time and allows you to focus on the important stuff.

**Balance** – in Paul's words, 'it's only work'. He also emphasised the importance of having outside interests, particularly in sport.

## Perspective

You need to take time off regularly, whether it's short breaks or a long holiday somewhere. This 'decompression time' is really important to mental and physical wellbeing. Susan Wojcicki, the CEO of YouTube, says:

'I think it's very important to take time off, and I've also found that sometimes you get really good insights by taking time off, too.'

Taking time out can help to cultivate a sense of perspective about your work/life balance, and can help see work-related problems and challenges as part of a wider picture. Sir Richard Branson (Chairman of Virgin Group) says:

'If I lost the whole Virgin empire tomorrow then I'd just go and live somewhere like Bali. Now if there was a problem with my family, health-wise, that's a problem.'

# Sport and performance in business

A lot of executives use sport as a way of keeping their minds and bodies fit and healthy and ready for optimum performance in the office or board room. Lord Sugar plays a lot of tennis. Paul Pester competes in triathlons, Peter Jones plays tennis, and Condoleezza Rice plays golf. Harriet Green, the recent CEO of Thomas Cook, sees a personal trainer four times a week and lifts kettle-bells as part of her sessions. She also practices yoga, and says this about prioritising time for exercise and wellbeing:

'If you can't do something for yourself for an hour a day, you have become a slave.'

Given there is still gender inequality in senior positions, a sports background could serve female executives very well. Results of a study released in October 2014 by the EY Women Athletes Business Network and espnW revealed that the majority of female executives surveyed said a sports background can help accelerate a woman's leadership and career potential, and has a positive influence on hiring decisions. It seems that the attributes to become successful in sport are easily transferable to the boardroom or corporate environment. Of the women in the EY survey, 53% said they still played sport as they moved into their working lives, and most still used sport to help them unwind. 37% said they felt it helped then to concentrate and focus on their work (swimming and running being the most popular activities).

Sport provides the opportunity to hone key skills that translate easily into business, and is also a great way to relax and de-stress. Executives are now encouraged to train themselves in the same way a professional athlete would by ensuring they are fit and sharp, and fully prepared to perform at the peak of their abilities.

## CASE STUDY: Ker Tyler

Ker Tyler is the CEO of a company called Fit for Leadership Ltd, which works with leadership teams and is dedicated to improving their individual and collective performances. Ker worked for a number of large financial institutions up until he suffered from burnout in 2007. This is his story.

I left the offices of the Spanish bank I was working for mid-afternoon one day. I felt claustrophobic, anxious and needed to just get away. I must have walked for a distance and suddenly realised I did not know where I was or what I was meant to be doing. I telephoned my partner in a state of panic and asked her where I was. Afterwards she told me of the terrible feeling of helplessness not knowing how to help or what to do. She actually contacted my daughter who lived in London but she could not determine where I was either, and felt equally helpless as I could not communicate rationally. We spoke and I became less stressed as she 'talked me down'. I continued to travel home shaken and shocked at my lack of personal control and not really knowing what had happened.

During this time, I was drinking too much coffee and far too much alcohol. I was short tempered and aggressive; suffered from a lack of quality sleep, and relationships with family and friends were breaking down. I had a poor diet and ate excessively, all of which got progressively worse. I had transformed from a positive, upbeat, fit, healthy and fun person to an introvert whose outlook was bleak. In addition, my weight had spiralled from a fit 16st 4lbs to an unfit and unhealthy 19st 13lbs (I am 6'5'). The final straw was waking up in bed at 4.00am and crying endlessly and not being able to stop. I felt like committing suicide and thought about it subsequently on several occasions.

During this period, my line manager called me into his office at 7.30am to formally ask me to leave the company. When challenged about why, he had no answers and smiled weakly. He lacked counselling skills, knowledge of anxiety, stress and depression and failed to enlist HR (who in the event were no better). The relief at being asked to leave was a big sign that I was very unhappy. In retrospect, I realise that my direct line managers both up and down did not know what to do or how to address the fact that I was clearly not 'right', even though ostensibly I was performing well and delivering the numbers. My employer was happy to see me go.

I went to see my GP. She was unavailable so I saw a locum. All she wanted to do was give me anti-depressants after measuring my state using a GAD (Generalised Anxiety Disorder) score which directed their solution. The GP wanted me out ASAP. I took the packet of drugs from the dispensary. I am proud and delighted to say that I had an epiphany and never touched one and never have. I appreciate for some they may work, for others less so.

I have always been competitive, and I've always been keen to please my parents, boss, colleagues, and be the best (whatever that is). My older brother was and is particularly clever and very successful in his field. He went to university – I did not. My younger brother who was following fast in my business footsteps died in a car crash, and unbeknown to me this had a deep and debilitating effect on my mental state. I felt weighed under by the feelings of loss and unfairness and couldn't understand why he had been taken. I now understand I failed to grieve properly and simply bottled up and carried the pain with me.

I was sporty and competitive; my older brother less so. I always wanted to prove my failure to go to university was not a barrier to my success. I measured everything in tangible things – big car, big house, and big salary. What has changed now is that my number one priority is my health – physical, mental and emotional. I now value meaningful relationships rather than shallow people who want you for all the wrong reasons.

After my burnout my family were great but found it very hard and I imagine I was hell to live with. The worst thing is the feeling of helplessness. It was not a case of stiff upper lip or pull your socks up; this was different and no one I knew had any experience of it. Early in the burnout process I'd got divorced and moved away from my children, friends and what had been home. My new partner was fantastic – caring, thoughtful and understanding but I wore her patience thin on many occasions! In the end I was paid redundancy. From being a high achiever, high earner, I became nothing. All new job applications were turned down, or I failed the interviews (which was unheard of previously). After twelve months, when I had spent my savings and the redundancy (high achievers tend to spend a lot and saving is always tomorrow), I decided to start my own business in a totally different area – helping others avoid what had happened to me.

I was ill-prepared for the change in every department. I will admit to having slipped back on a couple of occasions. In the process of setting up my own business from scratch, I allowed old habits around alcohol, poor food choices and lack of exercise to set me back. I tried throwing myself into an exercise regime, but my diet was bad and I thought I was fully well long before that was true.

Acceptance of the fact I was not well led me to seek relief in counselling, specifically Cognitive Behavioural Therapy. The CBT allowed me to understand what the issues were and how long I had been unwell, something that previously I had not been prepared to admit to myself. I made an effort to understand what burnout actually was, and realised that it was like any other illness. Suddenly I knew I could get well again; I could and would be OK. A big step forward for me was accepting that what I used to be like and what had happened in the past could not be changed, however I could change my future. It is now very important to me to live in the moment and learn to let go. I don't have to be in control, be number one or have stuff in order to be loved and cared for and to be happy.

My ego is still alive and well, so if I look in the mirror and ask myself, 'Am I good role model for my children and grandchildren, clients, friends and relatives?' and the answer is 'no', then I need to do something about it. The biggest challenge for me has been working through the massive amount of information that is out there and selecting the right thing for me mentally, emotionally and physically. I can't rely on willpower to make it work but need to find a way of changing myself permanently within my subconscious.

Deep down inside, everyone who suffers knows there is a problem – SEEK HELP! I am 100% sure that with the right support from professionals, good family support and with something to live for, there is a way out and it need not be torture. It is not something to feel guilty or bad about. You are not weak; you are strong just for accepting you have a challenge on your hands and then starting on the path to positive change.

Do not compromise your health. Happy and healthy beats rich and ill.

# 3. MENTAL AND PHYSICAL HEALTH

## Central Nervous System

The central nervous system is composed of the brain and the spinal cord, and can be considered the command and control centre of the human body. The central nervous system (CNS) communicates with the rest of the body via neurons linked to what is called the peripheral nervous system (PNS). When a stimulus is introduced to the body, receptors communicate with sensory neurons, which in turn communicate with motor neurons to effect a response within the CNS. Some of these responses could be called reflex responses, for example when your hand brushes close to a heated flame. The urge to pull your hand away from the heat is automatic, and happens outside of your conscious control.

Like any part of the body, the CNS can breakdown. A nervous breakdown (also known as a mental breakdown) can happen when the CNS is subjected to repeated and prolonged stress. It can also be caused by a chemical imbalance in the brain, usually linked to serotonin but also connected to noradrenaline, dopamine, acetylcholine and GABA (gamma aminobutyric acid). Worry, chronic stress, fear, anxiety, nervousness and panic attacks are all symptoms of a mental breakdown, and this is exactly what burnout is. You could say that burnout relates to the burned out nerves or synapses in the brain.

## Allostatic load

Allostasis is the process of achieving stability (homeostasis) through physiological or behavioural change. The female menstrual cycle is a good example; the body regulates itself by undergoing a period of change each month. An example of homeostasis is our core body temperature; our bodies maintain the same temperature by releasing or creating heat (sweating or shivering).

The term allostatic load was coined by Dr. Bruce McEwen, a professor of neuroscience at Rockefeller University. Put simply, allostatic load is the wear and tear on the body that develops over time when an individual is exposed to chronic and fluctuating stress levels. Interestingly, not all types of stress evoke the same response; it's the type of stress and how you deal with it that matters.

Every system in the body is affected by allostatic overload. Initially, the production of adrenalin and cortisol sharpen up the memory, keeping the individual focused in a time of danger. As the stress is repeated however, the neurons atrophy and memory becomes impaired. The immune system is impacted also; low levels of stress promote immune function by sending immune cells to the areas of the body where they are needed to defend against a pathogen. Chronic stress however, actually has the reverse effect by suppressing immune function, and the individual's risk of chronic disease suddenly becomes elevated.

## Stress and exercise

Stress is one of the biggest killers in today's society. Left unchecked it can lead to physical and mental breakdown, illness, the disintegration of families and relationships, the loss of jobs and livelihood, and in some cases loss of life. At best, it makes life difficult, more challenging and less enjoyable. Now exercise can't directly help certain things, like how to handle a difficult scenario at work, how to pay the mortgage, how to get your child into a good school or how to get a promotion, but it can help to improve your state of mind, help you sleep better and therefore think more clearly; it can help you think and communicate rationally and perhaps feel more relaxed and in control of other areas of your life. Exercise has been proven to decrease the production of stress-related hormones like cortisol, and increase the production of other hormones such as serotonin, adrenaline and dopamine, which together can contribute to making you feel more positive, happier and uplifted. There's also something very rewarding about making a plan of action, and then getting ready and going out and doing it, whether it's going for a run, completing an exercise session or just going for a walk. Just making a plan and sticking to it can be really gratifying. It can also help to take your mind off some of the negative emotions you might be experiencing, or give you some time out of the home or office.

## Anxiety, depression and exercise

Exercise is often under-prescribed by the medical community as part of a treatment plan for anxiety and depression, but despite that is widely considered to be central to helping people manage their condition. It isn't only the chemical responses in the region of the brain, (or specifically in the pituitary gland, which is not part of the brain but a small protrusion at the bottom of the hypothalamus), that help make people feel better about themselves, but also the physical changes that can help improve one's self-esteem and feelings of self-worth and competency.

## The brain and exercise

There are numerous positive changes to the brain that occur during and after exercise (in particular aerobic exercise). These changes occur in different parts of the brain, and in some cases the benefits are still enjoyed even after you stop exercising. These benefits include:

- Increased blood flow to the brain allowing it to thrive

- Adaptations that mean the brain can turn certain genes on and off, which can have the effect of boosting brain function

- Improved brain function can reduce the risk of diseases such as Alzheimer's, Parkinson's, strokes and cognitive decline

- Generation of neurotransmitters such as endorphins, dopamine and glutamate as well as encouraging the production of serotonin

- Supply of extra oxygen to a part of the brain called the hippocampus (responsible for learning and memory) which helps to create new brain cells. This process is called neurogenesis, and these new cells survive even after you stop exercising

## In contrast: the brain under stress

In the same way that our brains can be affected by exercise, they are also adversely affected by stress. Stress can be the trigger for harmful behaviours such as excess consumption of alcohol, cigarettes and prescription drugs, or poor sleep and hydration. Cortisol has been shown to damage and kill cells in the hippocampus, and there is robust evidence that shows it also causes premature aging.

## Sleep

Some people are blessed with the ability to fall asleep as soon as they hit the pillow, but the majority of clients I talk to have problems sleeping. Ideally, you should be getting seven to eight hours of good quality sleep, preferably uninterrupted, and in complete darkness. It's very important that the room you sleep in doesn't let light in, whether that's a street light, an LED on an alarm clock or television, a hall light or a night light. Sleep is inherently linked to diet and exercise, and put at its simplest, you aren't going to make good choices about food, or be energised or motivated to exercise (particularly at the early stages) if you're tired. If you use caffeine to combat tiredness, you'll also be relying on a stimulant to keep you going as well as raising your dehydration levels. The two go hand in hand: a good night's sleep translates to a better performance in the office or the boardroom, as well as other areas of life. Exercise also is a healthy way of expending energy, which in turn tires you out and enables you to sleep better, more deeply, and potentially gets you to bed earlier.

Research quoted recently in the *New Scientist* magazine could be good news if you have to deal with jetlag. Miho Sato and her colleagues at the Yamaguchi University in Japan have discovered that, in mice, the insulin released after a meal can restore a disrupted body clock. Apparently insulin can affect circadian rhythms, which in turn affects sleep, attentiveness and other functions, so it is possible to use food to influence insulin levels, and therefore our body clocks. Our central body clocks are reset daily by light, triggered by a part of the brain called the superchiasmatic nucleus. As well as our central body clocks, there are peripheral clocks in our cells and Miho Sato and her team believe that it is possible to adjust the schedule of these body clocks by eating. Should this prove to be true in human studies, it could be a game changer if you suffer from jetlag.

## Emotional eating

There is a definite link between anxiety, depression, feelings of low self-worth and eating, and this is not just symptomatic in over-eaters but in under-eaters also. If you don't feel good about yourself it's easy to make poor food choices, or to comfort eat, which is a fairly common response to bad news, stress, anxiety, low moods, or boredom. By putting more emphasis on diet and nutrition as part of an exercise plan, it can help to introduce a greater understanding of food and the impact it can have on our bodies and our ability to perform. This in turn can lead to better food choices, which can lead to improved sleep, which in turn leads to improved physical performance, and thus the cycle continues.

# Preventable diseases

The benefits of physical activity in preventing serious diseases are summarised in the table below:

| Condition | Role of physical activity |
|---|---|
| Overall mortality | Higher levels of regular activity are associated with lower mortality rates |
| Cardiovascular diseases | Regular physical activity decreases the risk of cardiovascular disease mortality, particularly coronary heart disease mortality |
| Cancer | Both the National Cancer Institute and Cancer Research UK strongly advocate physical exercise to help reduce the risk of all types of cancers |
| Osteoarthritis | Physical activity is not associated with joint damage or the development of osteoarthritis, but rather in those with osteoarthritis, exercise can reduce impairment and improve function |
| Osteoporosis | Weight-bearing physical activity can reduce the loss of bone mass typically associated with age |

| Falling | Physical activity and strength training can reduce the risk of falling in older adults |
| --- | --- |
| Obesity | Inactivity contributes to the development of obesity. Physical activity may favourably affect body fat distribution. Regular activity protects from cardiovascular disease, even in the absence of weight loss |
| Type II diabetes | Physical activity is recommended by doctors to patients with non-insulin-dependent diabetes mellitus because it increases sensitivity to insulin |
| Mental health | Physical activity appears to help relieve symptoms of depression and anxiety, and improve mood. It can also potentially reduce the risk of developing depression |
| Health-related quality of life | Exercise appears to improve the quality of life by enhancing psychological well-being and by improving physical function in persons compromised by poor health |

## Unexplained aches and pains

Medically unexplained symptoms can be quite common in people who are burned out or suffering from depression or chronic stress. Symptoms can include Irritable Bowel Syndrome (IBS), shortness of breath, trembling, chest pain, muscle aches, hot flushes, psychomotor agitation (restlessness) and low back pain. Often these symptoms can be distressing, because aside from the discomfort or pain they create, being unable to find a cause can be alarming. Usually there is something going on but at a deeper level that is causing these symptoms to appear. There is a direct link for instance between low back pain and depression; according to one study, major depression is thought to be four times greater in people with chronic back pain than in the general population (Sullivan, 1992).

Posture directly effects breathing. If you are in a slumped posture you compress your chest and therefore restrict how much your lungs can expand. Short and shallow breaths mean less oxygen is taken in to the body and poor removal of carbon dioxide. This in turn can lead to general aches and pains. Stress can manifest itself in your body in many ways, and often the first signs or signals will be physical. Interesting physical examples of extreme stress can include: jaw clenching pain, headaches, tremors, muscle spasm, insomnia, tiredness, weakness, fatigue, heartburn, stomach pain and difficulty breathing. Stress has been shown to result in individuals becoming more guarded and therefore physically tense. This can mean holding themselves in a protected posture with arms crossed, shoulders elevated, legs tucked under them and their trunk rolled into flexion. This sort of posture compresses internal organs. In turn this can reduce circulation which can cause muscle, joint and nerve pain.

## Self-medicating (alcohol, caffeine and nicotine)

If you are a smoker, the damaging and potentially fatal effects of smoking cigarettes or cigars are very well-documented and probably don't need repeating here. Should you happen to be in any doubt though, Google how smoking affects the respiratory system and that may put you off.

Consuming large quantities of alcohol damages just about every organ in the body, from the brain, to the stomach, to the liver. Some of the damage, for example to the brain, will be irreversible. Trying to function on a hangover not only puts strain on your heart, but the body will be working to get the toxins (the alcohol) out of the body rather than performing optimally. On an emotional level, cumulative and excessive alcohol consumption can lead to psychiatric problems, and contributes to depression and low self-esteem. Alcohol has a sedative-hypnotic effect, in other words it acts as a sedative that depresses activity of the central nervous system, and initially creates the impression of reducing anxiety and induces sleep, whereas the reality is the very opposite.

## Nutrition and a balanced diet

Following a balanced diet is absolutely essential for positive mental health, a healthy, lean body shape and a healthy, well-functioning heart. Optimal nutrition requires our diets to include fibre, vitamins and minerals (micronutrients) and food energy in the form of macronutrients such as carbohydrates, fats and oils, and protein. Each of these macronutrients take a bit of a bashing sometimes; fats have become associated with bad fat, weight gain, heart disease and obesity, whereas the reality is that whilst not all fats are good for you, some fats are essential to our daily diet. Balance is key. My belief is no diet should completely eliminate one of the macronutrient types completely; we need a balance of fats, protein and carbohydrates in our diet, combined with plenty of water and a good source of micronutrients.

Nutrition is often overlooked by people who have a very busy lifestyle. However, what you eat is absolutely vital to how you will perform, and what you look like, both on the inside and the outside. Food should be viewed as a fuel when it comes to exercising both your brain and the rest of your body. The commonly-used analogy is that of a car: in the same way that you wouldn't fill your car's petrol tank with toilet water and expect it to carry you sixty miles up the motorway, you can't expect diet coke and junk food to fuel your body through a 5K run, through a busy working week, or to give you the best chance of having a long and healthy lifespan. You get out what you put in. Begin by giving your body the nutrients it needs, and the right amount of calories, and you'll be amazed what it'll enable you to do in return. Ker Tyler, one of my case studies, uses the term Business Athlete, which I love. A professional (or even recreational) athlete wouldn't neglect any aspect of their nutrition or training, and it's the same for executives; if you want to perform well, you need to train well and stick to a plan.

## Weight management

Diets that drastically reduce what to eat are far less likely to work long term, and can have the opposite effect by making you store body fat by kicking in the body's starvation response, as well as potentially depriving your body of certain types of nutrients which are vital to its wellbeing. The starvation response can occur as a result of a sudden and dramatic reduction in calories consumed. The hormone leptin sends a signal to the hypothalamus in the brain that not enough energy is being ingested into the body. The hypothalamus responds by preserving the energy it has stored as fatty tissue, and at the same time begins to lower its daily calorie needs by reducing the volume of energy-hungry muscle tissue. So you start to consume muscle for energy, and store fat, which is counter-productive to most people's goals when dieting. This probably sounds really unhealthy to most people – that's because it is. It's also a very unpleasant way to try and lose weight; constant hunger combined with frustration at lack of results, or possibly even a weight gain.

Here are a few tips on what to look out for with your diet:

- Adopt a balanced diet which includes fresh fruit, vegetables, lean meats, dairy products and oily fish

- Check the ingredients of your breakfast cereal, and specifically the levels of salt and sugar. A lot of cereals are of low nutritional value so beware

- Eat whole grain toast rather than white bread, and avoid margarines which contain trans-fats and saturated fats. Use organic butter

- Cook meals using fresh ingredients rather than buying ready-meals or processed, pre-prepared foods

- Avoid refined carbohydrates such as white bread, white rice, white pasta, cakes, biscuits and pastries

- Drink plenty of water – aim for two litres per day

- Cut down on saturated fats and avoid hydrogenated fats where possible

- Don't skip breakfast – this is your most important meal of the day!

- Buy fresh, local, organic produce where possible

- Don't consume more than six grams of salt per day

- Avoid fizzy drinks – they can be full of sugar, additives and calories

- Moderate alcohol intake and drink water in-between alcoholic drinks

- Consider a multi-vitamin supplement – a lot of today's foods don't contain what we need in terms of daily vitamins and minerals; taking a daily supplement makes certain you've got what you need for the day

- Check and be aware of the sugar content of foods

It's worth saying a little more about sugar. There are often very high levels of sugar found in foods, especially processed (ready-meal) foods and in reduced fat or low-calorie options. Sometimes these sugars are concealed as additives like aspartame or Acesulfame K, which is just sugar by another name. You are often better off buying the full-fat option and having small helpings of it. A lot of people suffer from the 'sugar bounce', which are the highs and lows associated with sugar intake. It's well-known too that sugar also contributes to tooth decay, and contains 'dead' calories, which have no nutritional value.

There's a lot that can be said on this subject, but it's vital to appreciate that eating healthily isn't an option if you want to prolong your lifespan and improve your health. You can still love food whilst eating healthily, but be careful not to allow time – or more specifically, lack of it - to be an acceptable excuse for making poor food choices. You might need to plan ahead a little more, or walk a little further to find healthier food options, but it's definitely worth the investment in time.

## CASE STUDY: Rachel S.

I have known Rachel for over two years, both as a client and as a friend. Her story is a great illustration of how it's possible to ignore signs of chronic stress until eventually the body decides it's had enough. I think Rachel's story is inspirational as well as cautionary, and there's much in there for people to identify with.

I spent over fifteen years working in a high-pressure, deadline-driven environment. In the latter years I was based in Asia, handling multiple international projects, sometimes overseeing teams in up to three continents at a time. I frequently worked 12+ hour days, was constantly on flights and was regularly sleeping under six hours a night. Despite this hectic work environment, I felt as if I was enjoying my life. I believed that I thrived on the pressure, finding it hard to work without the buzz of a deadline, and I had a very active social life that I enjoyed, much of it revolving around bars. I took frequent trips and plenty of holidays. I thought that I had quite a good 'work hard, play hard' balance. I would have described myself as happy, and having a lot of fun.

Family and close friends would sometimes suggest that I was stressed but I didn't 'feel' stressed, which I took to mean feeling tense or uptight. Increasingly I did start to notice that I was exhausted on those weekends when I was able to take time out and that I felt a need to completely switch off on holidays. Although genuinely enjoying my work and my social life, I was not doing very much else. I was barely doing any exercise and was not taking part in anything that felt meaningful outside of work, blaming this on not having enough time.

In December 2007, I put my back out. One day I was fine, the next I couldn't get up from the bed without a great deal of pain, and very shortly after that I couldn't walk. It turned out that I had slipped a disc in my lower spine – a result of sitting too long, being too heavy and not exercising. My approach to life – work hard and then release by enjoying rich food, drink and late nights – was taking its toll.

I ended up in hospital for several weeks, eventually having surgery on my back. After my operation, the surgeon told me I was lucky not to lose the use of my leg because the pressure on my sciatic nerve had been so severe. There followed a long recuperation period; I was off work for around three months and then began by learning to walk at a normal speed again. Whilst the surgery was handled very well, there was little follow up other than some limited physiotherapy. I found that in terms of a full recovery, I had to take things into my own hands: finding a gym instructor for example, to help me start with some gentle exercise. I don't recall any medical professional talking to me about my overall lifestyle, stress or any mental health factors that might be linked to being in such bad physical condition. During this recuperation time I took a long hard look at myself and realised that despite my busy, fun life and apparently successful career, I was extremely unfit, overweight, tired and, as it turned out, quite literally broken.

With the benefit of hindsight, there were definitely warning signs that all was not well: in 2005 I had a very serious lung infection that put me in hospital for around two weeks and resulted in several months off work to recover. This may have been related to the fact that I was living in a highly polluted part of Asia, but my hectic lifestyle can't have helped. Instead of taking note and doing something fundamental to improve my health, as soon as I was well enough I not only went straight back to the same hectic lifestyle, but moved cities and took on a more challenging role.

Over the next couple of years I was sick numerous times. I had repeated bouts of flu, sinus infections, gastroenteritis and a kidney infection. I had also suffered from very poor digestion for years. Each time I was unwell I rested for a while, took medication and then carried on. Even when I wasn't sick I sometimes felt like I just needed to completely disengage and hibernate to recover from work and my social life. I put the illnesses down to air pollution and maybe working a bit too hard, but didn't stop to consider

# 4. THE HEALING PROCESS

A psychologist walked around a room while teaching stress management to an audience. As she raised a glass of water, everyone expected they'd be asked the 'half empty or half full' question. Instead, with a smile on her face, she inquired: 'How heavy is this glass of water?' Answers called out ranged from 8 oz. to 20 oz.

She replied, 'The absolute weight doesn't matter. It depends on how long I hold it. If I hold it for a minute, it's not a problem. If I hold it for an hour, I'll have an ache in my arm. If I hold it for a day, my arm will feel numb and paralysed. In each case, the weight of the glass doesn't change, but the longer I hold it, the heavier it becomes.'

She continued, 'The stresses and worries in life are like that glass of water. Think about them for a while and nothing happens. Think about them a bit longer and they begin to hurt. And if you think about them all day long, you will feel paralysed – incapable of doing anything.' **Remember to put the glass down.**

Successful recovery from burnout will usually involve several different healing techniques and strategies, depending on your starting point, what you enjoy, and what is appropriate at the time. The key aspects that I focus on within the Rise Method™ include:

- Exercise: empowering through movement
- Meditation
- Mindfulness and being present
- Relaxations techniques
- Yoga
- Laughter
- Power posing and posture
- Quiet time
- Strategies around social media
- Strategies around smart phones
- News ban

## Exercise: empowering through movement

It won't surprise you to read that exercise is the cornerstone of my Rise Method™. Appropriate levels of exercise and a healthy, balanced, tailored diet are vital to good health, and I strive to help my clients recognise that and learn to make those things part of their daily lifestyle.

Here are some of the main benefits that physical exercise brings:

**Mental health:**

- Generates endorphins (the 'feel-good' hormones)

- Generates norepinephrine (which can moderate the brain's response to stress)

- Generates dopamine (which can help rebalance you after other dopamine-dependencies)

- Boosts brain function by creating new brain cells (neurogenesis)

- Boosts creativity and prevents cognitive decline

- If outdoors, opens up access to fresh air and (potentially) increases levels of vitamin D3, melatonin and serotonin

**Physical health:**

- Healthy heart and lungs

- Strengthens muscles, tendons, joints and ligaments

- Increases energy

- Helps with weight management (even walking should not be underestimated)

- Improves posture

- Reduces risk of chronic diseases

- Improves sleep patterns and helps to retune circadian rhythms

- Generates feel-good hormones (see below)

## Cardiovascular benefits

Exercising regularly will induce changes to your cardiovascular system. 'Cardio' relates to the heart, and 'vascular' to the blood vessels, so cardiovascular benefits will therefore affect the heart and blood.

Predominantly aerobic training, such as circuits, jogging or boxing for example, will lead to an increased size of the heart (cardiac) muscle, which means your heart will be able to pump more blood around the body – this is known as increased cardiac output, defined as the amount of blood your heart can pump with each contraction multiplied by the amount of times it can beat per minute. Cardiac output improves significantly with increased fitness levels.

As mentioned before, your resting heart rate will come down as you get fitter. Your blood vessels will also become larger, and you will develop greater capillarisation, the net result of which will enable your body to carry more oxygen to the muscles when you exercise. After a relatively short period of regular exercise your blood pressure becomes lower, and you actually increase the volume of blood in your body too.

## Respiratory benefits

Exercising regularly helps increase the functional capacity of your lungs, so they become stronger and able to deliver oxygen into the bloodstream and remove carbon dioxide more effectively as you get fitter. Working aerobically for intense periods will specifically develop your lung capacity, and enable you to train for longer periods.

## Metabolic function

Your basal metabolic rate (BMR) will increase as you get fitter. BMR is the amount of calories your body consumes when you are at rest. So after an exercise session, whatever you're doing, you'll be burning more calories while you are sitting still than you would have prior to exercising. In essence, your body becomes more efficient whilst at rest which is great, but it also becomes more efficient whilst exercising. You will also reduce body fat more efficiently, and decrease the risk of developing insulin resistance and improve your glucose tolerance – vital for the prevention of type II diabetes.

## Muscular changes

Aerobic, as well as strength training, will develop improved muscle tone depending on what you want to achieve. Lifting weights, or resistance training as it's usually termed, can help strengthen your ligaments and tendons, and significantly improve your bone density and bone strength. This helps ward off conditions associated with getting older such as osteoporosis. There are also positive neural and biochemical factors associated with resistance training.

# Meditation

Quite often when I start working with executives who have experienced burnout, the concept of meditation can seem quite alien to them, and many think it's impossible. This is part of the problem of burnout; the body doesn't know how to shut off or settle down. Practising mediation is quite simply learning to be still, to be quiet and to allow the body time to restore itself back to homeostasis and a place of calm. There are a lot of preconceptions about meditation and what it means; I was very dismissive of it when I first came across it, thinking this wasn't something I had time for or needed. The truth is, everyone would benefit from meditating, even if it's only for ten minutes a day. The other misconception about meditation is that it involves being guided through a twenty minute dream-like state, or sitting in the Buddha position, or falling into a trance imagining yourself swimming with dolphins.

Meditating to me is about taking some time, even just a few minutes, and spending it thinking about nothing else but your body and what's going on. Your mind should be still, your thoughts should be boxed away, and the best way to start is to focus on your breathing. I was on a sales training day many years ago, and the sales director asked us all to sit in silence for several minutes and then make a note of the noises we could hear. Almost everyone came back with the same noises; passing traffic, pedestrians talking on their phones, the sounds of footfall on the pavement, the creaking of chairs, clothes rustling, and so on. No-one in the room (there were over 100 people there) said they heard the sounds of their breathing, despite it being the closest noise to them. This is because it's something that we do automatically, and therefore we don't hear it. What meditating does is bring your attention back to your breathing, and to allow you to focus on yourself again. In the same way that none of the salespeople in the meeting noticed their breathing because they were focusing externally on the white noise around them, if you're focusing on your breathing you automatically block out the white noise around you so you can fully focus. When asked about meditation and mindfulness, Steve Jobs of Apple said this:

'If you just sit and observe, you will see how restless your mind is. If you try and calm it, it only makes it worse, but over time it does calm... Your mind just slows down, and you see a tremendous expanse in the moment. You see so much more than you could see before.'

I also find reading in a quiet area can be very restorative, mentally. Just lying down and closing your eyes can also work. It's all about quietening the mind and taking some time to consider how you're feeling; the where, when and how isn't important, as long as you can disconnect from the outside world. It's not uncommon to see sportspeople meditating and going through visualisation exercises while waiting to come onto the court, pitch, athletics field or enter the ring. This in spite of the noise around them. Try it.

To some degree, all forms of meditation activate the 'relaxation response', a term originally used by the Harvard cardiologist Dr. Herbert Benson. The relaxation response is the opposite of the stress response, and describes the effects an activity or state of being have on the parasympathetic nervous system. The parasympathetic nervous system controls our basic processes of rest and digestion, and maintains homeostasis. This is the system that reduces the respiration and the heart rate; reduces the metabolic rate; decreases the production of stress-related cortisol; increases blood flow to the brain, and increases activity in the left frontal cortex which can strengthen the immune system and increase feelings of happiness. Through the practice of concentrated and committed meditation, you can enjoy all those benefits in exchange for ten to twenty minutes of your day. Now imagine a time when you felt most stressed, anxious or run-down; if I could offer to alleviate those thoughts and feelings, or even reduce them by 30% in exchange for twenty minutes of your time and a willingness to fully focus, would you take me up on my offer? That's what meditation could do for you.

## Mindfulness and being present

Mindfulness has become a buzz term recently, and there are many courses you can go on which teach you how to be mindful. Mindfulness isn't just about being aware, it's about being *fully aware* and in the moment. I often find myself 'in self' and thinking about something else when I'm going through the motions of doing something. It's very easy to find my thoughts drifting back to the past or ahead to the future; being present and being mindful will require you to consciously live in the here and now. The following excerpt is taken from Arianna Huffington's brilliant book, *Thrive*:

'Mindfulness is not just about our minds but our whole beings. When we are all mind, things can get rigid. When we are all heart, things can get chaotic. Both lead to stress. But when they work together, the heart leading through empathy, the mind guiding us with focus and attention, we become a harmonious human being. Through mindfulness, I found a practice that helped bring me fully present and in the moment, even in the most hectic of circumstances.'

More and more companies are recognising the need to protect their employees from stress. Perhaps unsurprisingly, Google was one of the first companies to value their employee's health in tangible ways; employees of all levels have been able to sign up for a mindfulness programme called Search Inside Yourself since 2007. Google also have walking meditations and mindful lunches which are available to all employees, not just senior executives. eBay and The Huffington Post have dedicated meditation rooms for all their employees, and the Bank of England experimented with 'working life seminars'.

Andy Puddicombe is the co-founder of an app called Headspace, which is a smartphone app that offers its users a simple and easy-to-use meditation technique to help improve physical and mental wellbeing. He has been asked to work with firms such as Credit Suisse, KPMG and Deloitte. He says:

'When we're happier and healthier, we're more productive. Collaboration and relationships are stronger. Creativity is boosted too, and every organisation relies on innovation. '

A UCL study, done in collaboration with one of the world's largest tech companies and a pharmaceutical company, showed a reduction in stress in diastolic blood pressure with the daily use of the Headspace app.

I heard someone say recently that taking executive and employee wellbeing seriously will become a major differentiator for firms in the future. Arianna Huffington said in a blog post:

'This is a tough economy. Stress reduction and mindfulness don't just make us happier and healthier, they're a proven competitive advantage for any business.'

More and more companies are now looking to recruit the top talent by restructuring their packages into lifestyle packages rather than concentrating solely on the financial rewards. A company that offers flexible working hours and locations, provides mindfulness programmes, includes opportunities to exercise during the working day and has a robust set of company policies that encourage a balanced working life will be able to differentiate itself from the competition.

Encouragingly the trend seems to be heading away from who can pay more and towards the kind of lifestyle benefits on offer. The recruitment and workplace review website Glassdoor recently published research that says happiness tends to round off at a salary figure of £55k/annum; after that, more money just results in diminishing returns in terms of happiness. Increasingly it would seem people are evaluating the pros and cons of running their own business and many are deciding it's worth the risks; statistics released by the Office of National Statistics (ONS) in August 2015 revealed that self-employment is now higher than it has been in the last forty years.

In America, companies offering meditation and other well-being programmes to their employees can in some instances enjoy lower healthcare bills. It seems that the clever thinking is now centred on creating a working environment for executives that is supportive and balanced. Offering meditation and mindfulness programmes and providing an environment which enables executives to stay healthy, will ensure that they can stay resilient, which is ultimately more important than the willingness to work long hours or sacrifice their health to drive forward results.

It's not just corporates that are starting to wake up to the idea of mindfulness as being a part of success and optimal performance. A lot of athletes are also incorporating it into their training.

Novak Djokovic is (at the time of writing) the number one tennis player on the men's circuit. He pays an incredible amount of attention to every single aspect of his training and preparation, not just his on-court training and gym work. He spends a lot of time thinking about his nutrition, (he is of the biggest advocates of the gluten-free diet), preparing his body with ice treatments, massage and physiotherapy, and following a highly disciplined regimen with regard to his sleep and hydration. After winning his second US Open title in September 2015, he said:

'I have always valued the care for my body and my mind and had this holistic approach to life. I always thought this is of the utmost importance for my tennis.'

He also dedicates a lot of time to considering how to prepare himself mentally. Tennis matches are won and lost in the mind, as is the case with most sports, and indeed with a lot of things in life. Have you ever lost a pitch or not got a job that you know you can have delivered on? Sometimes we sabotage ourselves mentally, and lose out on opportunities we should be winning. To help prepare himself for success, Djokovic is a big proponent of mindfulness. In his book, *Serve to Win*, he writes:

'I realised just how much negative energy I had coursing through my brain. Once I focused on taking a step back and looking at my thoughts objectively, I saw it plainly: a massive amount of negative emotion. Self-doubt. Anger. Worries about my life, my family. Fears about not being good enough. That my training is wrong. That my approach to a coming match is wrong. That I'm wasting time, wasting potential. And then there are the little battles: the imaginary arguments you have with people you won't even see that day over subjects that will never come up.'

Djokovic isn't the only person who is using meditation to differentiate himself:

'Meditation more than anything in my life was the biggest ingredient of whatever success I've had.' (Ray Dallo, billionaire founder of the world's largest hedge fund Bridgewater Associates)

'It's almost like a reboot for your brain and your soul. It makes me so much calmer when I'm responding to emails later.' (Padmasree Warrior, CTO at Cisco Systems)

'I walked away feeling fuller than when I'd come in. Full of hope, full of contentment, and deep joy. Knowing for sure that even in the daily craziness that bombards us from every direction, there is – still – the constancy of stillness. Only from that space can you create your best work and your best life.' (Oprah Winfrey, Chairwoman and CEO of Harpo Productions, Inc., after meditation in Iowa)

'If you have a meditation practice, you can be much more effective in a meeting. Meditation helps develop your abilities to focus better and to accomplish your tasks.' (Robert Stiller, CEO, Green Mountain Coffee Roasters Inc.)

Other well-known executives who are starting to wake up to the idea of mindfulness include Rupert Murdoch of News Corp, Marc Benioff of Salesforce.com and Bill Ford of the Ford Motor Company.

Professor Steve Peters is a renowned sports psychiatrist who has worked with snooker player Ronnie O'Sullivan, the senior men's football team at Liverpool and cyclists Victoria Pendleton and Sir Chris Hoy, amongst others. He has written a brilliant book which I often recommend to clients called *The Chimp Paradox*. He uses similar techniques for working with athletes and getting the best out of their performances.

## Relaxation techniques

There are different ways to relax, and what works for one person will differ from what works for another. Experiment with different ways; try having a bath, going for a walk or practising breathing exercises. Find something that relaxes you and then ensure it becomes part of your daily schedule. Perhaps surprisingly, it might be a sport that relaxes you. I think this is good, if it allows you to shut off. The important thing is that it isn't stressful. If your chosen sport is boxing, or you are fiercely competitive, then perhaps this isn't the ideal form of exercise (at least not in the context that I'm talking about here).

# Yoga

I discovered yoga a few years ago, having previously allowed my preconceptions of it to blind me to its many benefits. My view was changed when I began doing weekly yoga classes with a local teacher Ellie who is now part of my team. Not only is it very relaxing, but it also helps strengthen and calm the body, as well as including lots of long, deep stretches which many people really need. Most executives are very time-crunched, and even for those who do manage to exercise, a lot of their time will be spent sitting at a desk or in a car. Prolonged sitting is very damaging for the body, and can result in tight muscles and connective tissue; shortened hamstrings, tight hip flexors, rounded shoulders and a kyphotic spine (curved upper back) are commonly seen. A sixty or ninety minute yoga session can address those issues, and leaves the body feeling tinglingly good about itself.

I asked Ellie what impact she thought yoga has on chronic stress:

'There are many reasons why yoga can be of benefit if you are suffering from (chronic) stress. The combination of focusing on the asanas (postures) and breathing anchors us in the present moment. There is no space in the mind for thoughts to drift off to "worry" if you are on the mat, focusing on holding your warrior pose. During a yoga session there is a lot of emphasis on the breath – sometimes taking deeper breaths down into the tummy and controlling the exhale or just being aware of your breathing helps to calm the mind. A yoga session can make you more aware of your body and your emotions and the awareness and acknowledgement of stress can be the first step in helping to control it.'

One of the challenges I had when I started yoga is learning to relax and quieten the mind. It's the same with my clients; those who need it most often don't think they can make time to lie still, relax or spend an hour stretching. Part of my role is to challenge that thinking and encourage clients to give it a try. Ellie agrees:

'To give yourself full permission to do nothing at all but lie down and relax can be a huge challenge as we are so well trained to be constantly doing something, or more usually numerous things all at once. We check our emails while cooking dinner, while thinking about what to wear to work the next day, while wondering what to get our friend's daughter for Christmas – all at once. So asking yourself to do nothing, asking the body to be still and the mind to stop thinking can be really difficult. But, like everything else, even relaxation gets better with practice.'

If you are burned out then learning to work with your breathing and giving yourself time away from the rest of the world to fully relax can be of huge benefit.

# Laughter

There are several different areas of the brain which are responsible for different functions. The limbic system is involved in all our emotions, including laughter, and some of the other more basic functions required for survival. If one aspect of the brain is disrupted or isn't functioning properly, serious problems can ensue. It's the amygdala and the hippocampus which are the two limbic structures that are activated when you laugh. Aside from activating your stress response, which has been discussed already, laughter can soothe tension, and stimulate your organs by enhancing your intake of air. Laughter improves your mood, and can be a great way to connect with other people. Think back to when you last really enjoyed a good laugh; it might seem like quite a long time ago. Try watching something on television that used to make you laugh, or reminisce with an old friend and see what it does for your mood.

The link between the mind and body is well-known, and often pain in the body can be linked back to your emotional state of wellbeing. Rebecca van Klinken is a physiotherapist, and a lot of the patients she sees in her clinic are suffering from stress in one form of another. Often they come in to see her with unexplained pain, and she thinks this is down to extreme stress.

'Pain which can be linked with emotional state of wellbeing tends to be very widespread. In other words, clients complain of it moving around their body from joint to joint or muscle to muscle. Clinicians often diagnose these people with fibromyalgia or Chronic Fatigue syndrome. The cause of either of these diagnoses is unknown but in a lot of cases it happens to individuals who have been through a stressful ordeal of some sort.'

## Power posing and posture

Posture can be negatively affected by stress, and poor posture can result in injury and pain. Research done by Elizabeth Broadbent, Ph.D. of the New Zealand University concluded:

'There are physiological links between our brains and our bodies so that certain muscle positions can affect the functioning of our nervous and endocrine systems. Sitting upright allows the nervous system to respond to the stressor better.'

In an article in the *Journal Health Psychology*, a researcher said:

'Sitting upright may be a simple behavioural strategy to help build resilience to stress.'

Another study conducted at Harvard University (Cuddy, 2012) found a distinct correlation between the stress hormone cortisol and the posture (or power poses). Cortisol levels decreased when an individual had adopted a high power pose (in other words a relaxed pose), and increased after they had adopted a low power pose (tensed). Researchers also found that when an individual has feelings of power and self-control, this can boost testosterone levels and reduce cortisol.

We know that body language can have a profound effect on stress levels. Our non-verbal communication can also have a very strong influence on how we are perceived by others. Take this a step further, and you can see this could also be a determinant of future success, both personally and professionally. In a very interesting TED Talk originally shown in June 2012, Amy Cuddy discusses the relationship between power posing and hormone levels (testosterone and cortisol), and argues that your body language shapes who you are and has a profound influence on the decisions you make. This is taken from a transcript of her talk. View it online here: http://www.ted.com/talks/amy_cuddy_your_body_language_shapes_who_you_are/transcript?language=en):

'So this is what we find. Risk tolerance, (Cuddy is referring here to gambling), we find that when you are in the high-power pose condition, 86% of you will gamble. When you're in the low-power pose condition, only 60%, and that's a whopping significant difference. Here's what we find on testosterone. From their baseline when they come in, high-power people experience about a 20% increase, and low-power people experience about a 10% decrease. So again, two minutes, and you get these changes. Here's what you get on cortisol. High-power people experience about a 25% decrease, and the low-power people experience about a 15% increase. So two minutes lead to these hormonal changes that configure your brain to basically be either assertive, confident and comfortable, or really stress-reactive, and feeling sort of shut down. And we've all had the feeling, right? So it seems that our non-verbals do govern how we think and feel about ourselves, so it's not just others, but it's also ourselves. Also, our bodies change our minds.'

## Quiet time

Allocating part of the day to quiet time is also vital. This might be five or ten minutes spent reading in bed at the beginning or the end of the day, or it might be spent sitting in your car before heading into the office or home. Just having a few moments to gather your thoughts can make an appreciable difference to how you feel. If you can combine this with breathing exercises, particularly if you feel your stress levels rising, you'll be doing yourself a big favour. Try and shut off from the outside world, both mentally and literally – no news, no television, no radio, no phones!

## Social media

Facebook. Twitter. Pinterest. Instagram. LinkedIn. Social media has a place, but it's increasingly taking up more and more of our time. Facebook now has over 1.5 billion users who log in at least once a month. Towards the end of August 2015, for the first time over a billion people used Facebook on a single day. That's one in seven people on planet earth. Checking for updates or responding to updates has become an intrinsic part of our hourly lives. These applications want you to be operating within them and communicating, posting, liking or tweeting, and so they are designed to lure you in and keep you coming back – again and again and again. Have you ever thought about why this is? It's partly down to dopamine.

A number of studies have been done to look at the relationship between happiness and Facebook usage, and loneliness and Facebook usage. One meta-analysis by Hayeon Song and her team from the University of Wisconsin-Milwaukee looked at this extensively in a study called *Computers in Human Behaviour*. They concluded that there was a connection between Facebook and loneliness, but that Facebook didn't make people lonely; lonely people were more likely to be drawn to Facebook. As Song says:

'Does spending so many hours with a machine keep people from making real connections with other people? Or, does it allow people who are shy or socially awkward a chance to connect with others in a way that's more comfortable for them than face-to-face communication?'

There are strong arguments on both sides of this debate, but I do think that all forms of social media have a time and a place. Spending too long staring at a screen or interacting with others online isn't necessarily a good use of time, and isn't always that social either. Song concludes:

'Facebook is so widespread, and it's evolving. For some people, it is almost like an addiction because they become so deeply involved. That's why it's important to understand the causes and the long-term consequences of using social media.'

## Smart phones

Smart phones, Blackberry devices and other portable devices now enable us to stay connected to the outside world on a continual basis. Twenty-four hours a day, for seven days a week, we are able to access news, market data, email, text messaging, social media and just about any website we like with a few taps or swipes of an index finger. Never have we had access to so much information, so quickly. I attended an event recently in the City where I heard the results of a survey asking people what made them stressed at work and how they coped. One survey respondent said the game changer for them was email; they summarised by saying that email makes things relentless. Some companies will have policies around email and response times outside of business hours, but most don't, or if they do it's not enforced.

I worked for a company which had a policy written into the handbook stating that employers were not allowed to contact an employee during pre-booked vacation time; this wasn't always respected but generally it was, and it's certainly a start. The reality is there is an expectation now that executives will be available when needed. Most people I know, if not all, frequently check their mobile or Blackberry outside of business hours. I have done this, and I can't recall one example of when I've checked my email and was glad I did. I can however recall several occasions when I've seen an email that I'd preferred not to have seen until Monday.

Most contracts for banks, law firms or accountancy firms will have a clause that waives the employee's rights to the European Working Hours Directive. In a survey of respondents coordinated by the Priory Group and taken from their website, 96% said they worked more than their contracted hours; 41% felt the need to reply to a personal text or social media message, and 58% they felt more stressed than they did a year ago. One in four people said they worked more hours because they felt it was expected of them.

Setting yourself rules for your phone and email is a critical priority. You cannot control your mental or physical state if you're being manipulated and controlled by the messages coming into your phone. Some of these rules might include:

- establishing 'no-go' times when your phone is off – for example before 8am or after 8pm

- letting staff or managers know that you're unavailable in these times – either verbally or using an auto-reply message

- have a separate phone for personal email, calls and messages (but apply the same rules around usage at the beginning and end of the day)

- delete icons for apps that waste your time, such as Facebook, Twitter, and any others (you can still access the sites from a PC but this will prevent you from wasting time looking at content that excites the monkey-brain part of your mind and stops you focusing on you)

- delete apps that have alerts (even news sites like the BBC) or turn off the alerting service

- keep your phone in the other room, especially at night (if you use it as an alarm clock then keep it on the other side of the room so that you aren't tempted to check it in the night or end up reading from it before you go to sleep)

- get in the habit of going out without your phone on weekends or some evenings; you'll miss it to start with and will have several panicky 'where's my phone' moments but after a while you'll start to appreciate what's going on around you without the distraction of a mobile phone

- allocate specific times of day for checking, replying or creating emails and messages – if you're disciplined about this then you'll probably increase your productivity as well as reducing your stress levels

- be realistic about setting expectations in terms of your response times – if you inform people that you only check emails or messages every morning for an hour, they won't have the expectation that you'll respond quickly to an email

- I have heard of people who ask guests to leave their phones and Blackberry devices by the front door when they arrive for a dinner party – this is a great idea and ensures everyone is free of their number one distraction (and means unexpected photos don't pop up in your timeline the next day!)

## News ban

I like to encourage my clients to avoid reading or watching the popular news channels whilst we begin the process. Most of the popular media channels, by which I mean television, newspapers and the internet, don't have positive stories to report. Most of the news items are about war, famine, struggle, despair, loss, and quite a lot of drama too. What underpins all these themes and stories is this: fear. I like my clients to try and put all that to one side whilst we go through the Rise Method™. I don't insist on it, but mostly it just serves as a distraction, with no upside.

At a time when you might be struggling with your self-esteem, unable to think rationally and clearly, and perhaps dealing with financial pressures and relationship issues, you can live without knowing what's going in the news. Whilst stories about the conflict in Syria and world famine are tragic, when you're burned out, you are not in a position to deal with any of that. Sadly, these issues will still be there when you're recovered, and you can consider then what you can do to help.

# 5. MY STORY

I became interested in helping people recover from burnout because I came very close to it myself. I resigned from my job as an Account Director in the City in March 2012 in less than ideal circumstances, but I had no regrets about doing so then and I certainly don't have any now.

I come from a family background that was loving, but quite turbulent. My parents divorced when I was quite young, and my brother and I lived with our mother. Mum worked as a PA, and my father ran his own businesses. He was my idol growing up as I wanted to run companies and do what he did. I wasn't traditionally academic, and in fact was a pain at school. I preferred pushing the boundaries of what I could get away with, making people laugh and doing the bare minimum than actually getting on with any work. This carried on until I had completed my GCSE's and had to apply for the Sixth Form. I thought I'd scraped by with enough GCSE's to get entry into Sixth Form, but in the end that didn't turn out to be the issue. It transpired that whilst I wanted to stay on, the powers-that-be didn't want me; I was politely but firmly asked not to bother applying.

After much discussion with both my parents, we decided that I should try and get into the local girl's grammar school. Much to everyone's surprise, they accepted me into their Sixth Form. Unbeknownst to me at the time, the year I entered (1992) was the first year they began the grant-maintained status, so more pupils equalled more money. Hence I was admitted, along with several other misfits who ordinarily wouldn't have got anywhere near the school gates. My days there were short-lived however, and I was asked to leave in the first few months as a result of disruptive behaviour and generally not fitting the profile of a grammar school girl.

Fortunately for me, my mum, along with a few of my teachers, took up the cause on my behalf and I was readmitted on the basis that the formal process wasn't followed by the Headmistress (who in a strange twist of fate was dismissed from her post by the board of governors for malpractice a few weeks afterwards). With her off my back, I was able to get my head down and I left the school in 1994 with three A-levels. University followed, a thoroughly enjoyable although hedonistic three years spent reading English Literature in Bangor, North Wales.

Despite being very popular, I never really felt that I fitted in. That was when I learnt to blend in and be a social chameleon, which is a useful skill in sales but has its drawbacks. I also was quite self-reliant, and had conditioned myself to internalise thoughts and feelings rather than share them with others.

I wasn't able at that stage of my life to be authentic about who I was, and when I discovered alcohol around the age of seventeen, I found a way to express my feelings, but these feelings would often manifest themselves in anger. Alcohol was to become a major part of my life for the next twenty years, and I often used it to suppress and express aspects of my personality.

A young adult who uses alcohol as a substitute for relying on other people can encounter problems later in life when they experience challenges or go through difficult times. How we respond to our problems and struggles when we're young is likely to be the way we deal with these things as an adult, and this is one of the reasons that alcohol abuse and alcoholism develops. Add to this the inability to express who you are, and you have the potential for destructive behaviour. I'm sure you know of at least one person who is either concealing an important aspect of their character, living a life they don't enjoy, or are stuck in a job they hate. They spend their time doing something that doesn't reflect their own personal values or allow them to express themselves. This is a major reason why people burnout.

My sales career began in 1997 when I took a job as an Account Executive for a large Canadian software company. I loved the role, and really enjoyed throwing myself into something that came easily. I worked at other companies in a similar industry sector after that, and always in similar roles but a grade or two up from the last one.

Sales is a very sociable career choice; there are a lot of nights out with suppliers, distributors and resellers, and of course customers. I found that I tended to be allocated the more sociable clients, so I often found myself going out with customers who really wanted to enjoy themselves. I also enjoyed this at the time, but as the years progressed, this was to work out less and less well for me. I also started to feel less attuned to what I did for a living; I enjoyed selling creatively, working on bespoke solutions for clients and bringing in business deals that were valuable to my company, but I also started to feel distanced from my colleagues.

There were a lot of aspects to corporate life that I felt removed from, such as the swagger and arrogance that can come with position and titles rather than achievements. I also felt constrained by the style of clothing (suits and heels), which wasn't and isn't really me. I struggled with being desk-based too; even though I spent a lot of time visiting customers as part of my job (there were targets for how many meetings you were supposed to do in a week), their offices might be ten minutes' walk from mine, so it wasn't an active role at all. All of this was making me feel hemmed in, and I started to rely more on alcohol to relieve these feelings.

Fast-forward to 2012, and my abrupt resignation from my last job at a market data company in the City. A combination of very heavy alcohol intake, boredom and a lack of fulfilment, and a realisation that I no longer cared about my chosen career was making me very frustrated and unhappy. The frustration and boredom was driving the drinking, which was impairing my ability to perform. This led to poor results, which resulted in heightened scrutiny of my movements and sales figures. All of this became self-perpetuating, cranking up the pressure which in turn led to more drinking. This had been going on for years, but I was very good at concealing what was really going on, and was functioning highly.

This ability to function in the face of inner chaos is probably one of my biggest strengths but also biggest weakness, and in the end I was very close to burned out by the time I took action. I resigned from my job on Friday night, and negotiated a period of one month's gardening leave to be taken immediately. By this point I was drinking very heavily, and for most of the waking day. Things had spiralled completely out of control.

It was only by hitting this rock bottom that I was able to give myself the opportunity to review where I was at in my life. The warning signs had been there for some years. During a very stressful time in my career, I can recall having a very heavy night of drinking quite early on in the week, and the next day I felt very unsettled and anxious. The hangovers had changed in nature from what one might consider the standard nausea and headache to very anxious and shaky. I know now that this is one of the first signs of physical addiction.

I went into work quite early (this was part of my strategy of trying not to stand out when I felt like this), and was due at a meeting at a client's offices later that morning. I had several espressos before the meeting to wake myself up. During the meeting, I began to feel very strange, and my hands started trembling and then shaking quite badly. I had been taking notes whilst my colleague and I talked to the client, but I had to stop because of the shaking. My heart was racing and I was sweating. The room we were in was making me feel even worse as it was windowless and I felt very claustrophobic. My throat was very dry and I was desperate for some water, but despite having some in front of me, I didn't dare to lift the cup in case I spilt it by shaking. I'm still not quite sure how I made it through the meeting. Afterwards in the lift, I explained to my colleague that I had to go home as I didn't feel well.

I took the rest of the day off and visited the doctor who signed me off for one week and cited anxiety due to stress as the reason. That was my opportunity to make some changes but I chose not to, and returned to work after just a week. My anxiety in work situations worsened and I often struggled to manage it. Preparing for meetings was a challenge, especially if I was attending with colleagues who I felt would notice the change in me. In the end I opted for the geographical cure. The geographical cure refers to the act of moving home or changing jobs in the hope that whatever you're trying to escape or fix goes away (it doesn't).

I moved jobs and started again at a new company but despite a bright start, the problems didn't really go away. All the things that were wrong – the alcohol, the lack of authenticity, the boredom, the lack of fulfilment, the disinterest – simply moved with me. Of course initially when you start at a new company, everything is just that – new. So you can fool yourself that this job is different, you'll be successful here, the people are great, the systems and processes are more efficient and the commission scheme is better and more lucrative. Inevitably, the old demons return and you find yourself feeling even more despondent as you realise nothing's changed.

I mentioned earlier in the book that we tell ourselves a million little white lies every day, and when you're heading for a burnout I think this is definitely true. I managed to ignore the elephant in the room for years; that alcohol was only ever going to sabotage my success and accelerate my decline into burnout. I ignored the fact that I didn't like what I did for a living (in the context in which I was doing it), and that in fact I had gone into this job because it's what I thought I should do and who I should be. It's pretence that will stifle happiness and success. It's that pretence that will cause unmanageable amounts of stress to build up inside you.

Ultimately accepting that things had to change was the first stage of the process that I have subsequently developed and now call the Rise Method™.

To begin with, I thought about what I needed to do to recover my energy and start working towards my full potential again. This process followed a basic framework, the first aspect of which was to review my lifestyle and evaluate where I was at the time. This required me to take a long hard look at why I had ended up where I had, and to clearly identify what aspects of my life were not serving me well anymore. Some of this was quite obvious to me; what had begun as a bit of fun, had developed into a psychological dependency, then a physical dependency and finally into full-blown alcoholism.

Aside from the alcoholism, I drank because I was bored, because I was not doing something that reflected my authentic self and I knew I was wasting my potential; in effect, I was suppressing my authentic self and not allowing it to thrive. In reviewing my old lifestyle, I identified the areas that I needed to work on, and as importantly, identified areas where I needed to find alternatives or new ways of doing things. The first and most obvious step was to go through the process of giving up alcohol so that I could think clearly, with no reliance on mind-altering substances to mask or cloud my judgement. I also thought about my job, and made a list of what was important to me and what my beliefs were (see Appendix A). To get this clarity, I wrote down a list of as many statements as I could think of that started with 'I believe'. Here are a couple of examples:

> I believe that exercise can be the most powerful mind-altering therapy there is

I believe in the wonders of the human body and
what it will do for you if you treat it with respect

I also wrote down as many statements beginning with the
words 'I do what I do because...' as I could think of. Again,
here are a couple of examples:

I do what I do because I want to build a business
based on what I love doing and wholeheartedly
believe in

Our bodies are meant to move so I spend my
time showing clients how to do this safely and
enjoyably in order to prolong their health span

I strongly urge you to go through this process; write down as
many things as possible and keep going until you either can't
think of anything else, or you get that light bulb moment
when your true purpose reveals itself to you, as it did to me.
It might be a bit too soon to start the 'I do what I do because'
process, but the 'I believe' exercise will be the best tool you
have in finding out what your true vocation is. I came to the
conclusion that several things were important to me:

- to perform a role that allowed me to help others

- to enjoy the autonomy of working for myself

- to set up my own business and give myself the challenge of seeing what I could build

- to help other people in my position

- to work outdoors as much as possible

- to create a business culture that prioritises health, fitness and wellbeing above all else

- to have a job that truly reflects my authentic self

- to create a business that thrives at the intersection of my two passions – personal empowerment and movement

The obvious move having established what was important to me, was to look into qualifying as a personal trainer and go about setting up my business. Bodyshot Personal Training was launched in May 2012: our only assets were my personal training qualification, a website, some basic equipment and most importantly, a well-thought through framework that I believed would help my clients to achieve balance in their lives. I am pleased and proud to say that what I do for a living now reflects who I am and what I believe in.

Having gone through the review process, I then worked out what I needed to do to re-ignite myself, and restore my good health. I looked at my eating habits, my levels of exercise, what I did to relax (nothing at that time), my stress levels, my life load, hydration levels, and so on. With some help, I also looked a bit harder at aspects of my personality in a bid to leave no stone unturned. By this I mean having someone ask me some difficult questions about how I managed stress, whether I asked for help, what thought processes I underwent in difficult times, and so forth. Was I a person to ask for help when I needed it? Did I share what was on my mind with anyone? Did I employ any mindfulness techniques to balance out stress? (The answers to these questions was always no). This can be a difficult part of the process as you will need to dig deep and face things you might have previously boxed away, but it is important. I was, and am still surprised, by how little I can remember about some things, and this is probably because I have always tended to 'archive' things that it suits me to forget. This has sometimes worked well for me but I wouldn't recommend it as an ideal strategy. You might wish to work with a counsellor or another professional at this stage, although going through the exercises I've mentioned is very helpful and can be done alone.

Part of the restore process for me was completely overhauling my diet. I had previously eaten ready meals (which I had bought from a high-end supermarket and therefore thought were high quality!), washed down with copious amounts of red wine. I used supermarket brand supplements (a multivitamin normally) and tried to buy foods that purported to be healthy from some of the upper end food stores when I was at work. (A note of caution; foods are often less healthy and more calorific than you might think). I began to take an active interest in nutrition, reading books on the subject and going on courses as well as throwing out the little I had in my kitchen and buying fresh, organic or spray-free produce either from the source itself or as directly as possible.

I started buying foods based on provenance not price, and took an interest in where it came from. 'Locally sourced and organic' has since become a catchphrase for me. I discovered a local not-for-profit scheme that delivers vegetables from organic or spray-free farms within a sixty mile radius of London; Google to see if there's a similar scheme in your area. This scheme ensures you get what's ready to come out of the ground, it's as fresh as it can be (in some cases it's still caked in earth!), the farmers get a guaranteed price, and there's minimal waste as nothing is rejected based on its unusual shape or size.

Abstaining from alcohol was obviously a big game changer, but introducing healthy, freshly-cooked foods of a much higher quality than before also meant my body shape was changing. I was about two-and-a-half stone overweight in May 2012, which came off at a healthy rate until my body found its natural set point, where my weight has stayed ever since. Taking an interest in nutrition is a crucial part of taking control of your health.

I had previously exercised about three to four times a week but was treading water in terms of weight management given my alcohol intake and unhealthy diet. As soon as I made those vital changes, my exercise output improved significantly and I got a lot more benefit from it mentally as well as physically. I've always enjoyed fairly physical forms of exercise such as boxing, tennis, and circuits, and as I got lighter and was able to put more into it, both my boxing and tennis improved.

The big gaps in my physical training were around three areas: there was nothing in my weekly regime that took into account the need for stretching and flexibility; there was nothing that gave me an opportunity to connect with how I was feeling through movement; and there was no relaxation built into my programme. I changed this by finding a yoga teacher (we met Ellie earlier in the book, who is now part of my company), and having weekly ninety-minute, one-to-one sessions with her at my house. This has been invaluable to me for working on stretching and flexibility, but also connecting with my body. Through yoga, I've been able to improve my fitness, as well as practice breathing exercises which are beneficial to me in terms of stress management, and also useful for my sport (especially boxing).

Breathing is an important issue in stress or anxiety disorders. If you breathe correctly (i.e. deeply to expand the base of the lungs and not risking overuse of the neck and upper chest muscles) you can reduce stress/anxiety levels. I also started having regular massages and frequently see an osteopath, both of which make sure that I'm able to operate at my physical peak at work and in my personal life. It might sound clichéd, but now I feel I have everything in my life that means I can shine again.

As well as changing and adapting the type of exercise I did, I tried to cycle instead of taking the train or driving, and generally was more active. Not having to sit at a desk for most of the day, five days a week, was a big benefit to my health too. I will say at this stage that it's important to ensure you are not doing too much exercise. One of the common characteristics of burnout is doing too much or being quite extreme, so just watch that you don't overdo the exercise. It's all about balance!

Once I started to recover, I gradually re-introduced a few things back into my routine. I thought of this as rebalancing, and a key part of that was making a checklist for myself that I could refer to in the future. This is really important, as it provides a way of making sure you aren't doing too much or slipping back into old habits. Close friends and family can be a good sounding board in this regard too; usually they will be the first to suggest if they feel you're heading backwards on something or some of the old personality traits are surfacing again. Listen to those people as chances are they've seen the iceberg before you have, as they have the benefit of an external viewpoint.

I'd say it took several months to recover, and some of the case studies would say longer. It's definitely a process, and there's no fixed timeframe. It takes as long as it takes, and you aren't the same person afterwards (and that's a good thing). You'll learn some valuable lessons, and will hopefully be able to live a more meaningful life in the future.

My company, Bodyshot, is now a team of six people and we have big growth plans for 2015 and beyond. We specialise in bringing the science of genetics to women's fitness, and have an online platform where clients can purchase a package of tests that tell them their ideal diet type and what type of exercise is best suited to them. The results and supporting documentation are then delivered in a follow-up consultation with one of my qualified coaches. It is our goal to become the specialists in genetics-based women's fitness in the UK.

We also have a brand called Recovery Fitness that helps clients suffering from stress, anxiety and depression; personally it gives me a great deal of satisfaction helping people restore their mental health, or better manage their conditions. Working with some of the Recovery Fitness clients helped prepare me for the burnout coaching, for which I am now known. In 2015, I decided to adapt the informal process that I'd followed for myself and formalise it into a concept that could be used to help others recover from professional burnout. In fact, it can also work for anyone who needs to make lifestyle changes, whether they be problems with drinking, smoking, weight management (that includes being underweight as well as overweight), anxiety, depression, unhappiness, or low self-esteem. The process is called the Rise Method™; more on this in Chapter 7.

TIP: Take a moment now to consider my story and see if you can identify areas where you can empathise with what I've said. Look for the similarities not the differences.

# 6. AUTHENTICITY OF SELF

What I hope you've realised by now is that burnout is very strongly linked to authenticity of self. I burned out because I wasn't doing something that was an authentic reflection of myself. Many others have burned out for the same reasons, across all walks of life and not just in the corporate world.

Take the example of Vicky Beeching, an English singer who studied theology at Oxford University before moving to the US to further her music career. Unless you lived in bible-belt America, or were a die-hard fan of American Christian music, you'd be forgiven if you hadn't heard of Vicky Beeching. At that time (2014), she was a hugely successful singer/songwriter, having released three studio albums, and was the poster girl for American Christians. Her public profile soared when in 2014, she controversially came out as gay. Unsurprisingly, this caused a lot of consternation in religious circles, and encouraged people everywhere to share their opinions, good and bad.

That isn't the story though. For years, because of her upbringing and the exclusively religious circles that she moved in, she believed that the feelings she had towards women were wrong, and should be suppressed at all costs. These feelings were reinforced in quite dramatic terms by the overwhelming majority of people around her. She has described being at a Christian youth summer camp where an exorcism was performed on her to try and cure her of her perversion.

In order to conceal these feelings, Beeching threw herself into her work, song writing and performing. In an interview with Patrick Strudwick for the Independent in August 2014, she said:

'I felt there was something so wrong with me, according to the Church, that maybe I could make up for it by getting good grades.'

Following her graduation, Beeching moved to the home of country music, Nashville, America, recorded three albums and performed endlessly. Inside though, she was hiding her true, authentic self, and eventually she burned out. In an interview with the *Independent Newspaper*, Beeching says:

"I was blow-drying my hair and looked in the mirror and noticed this white line down my forehead.'

It turned out that the scar was a sign of a very serious auto-immune condition called linear scleroderma morphea, or more specifically a form of the disease called *coup de sabre*. At its worst, large areas of the body can turn into scar tissue, and it can be fatal. Treatment was extensive chemotherapy. Beeching was shocked and flew home to the UK as soon as she could.

Once back in the UK, she consulted a doctor who suggested the cause might be mental; he encouraged her to consider whether there was a trauma or point or stress which might be causing her to be deeply unhappy. For Beeching, it was obvious; suppressing her sexuality was the root cause. She says:

'I looked at my arm with the chemotherapy needle poking out, I looked at my life, and thought, I have to come to terms with who I am." She publically came out in 2014 to a predominantly supportive public, although there was some pushback from certain areas of the Church.

To deny your sexuality is to deny authenticity of self. To deny any aspect of your true self means you cannot and will not live a happy, fulfilled, focused and successful life. If you've burned out, one of your top priorities must be to find a way to make peace with your authentic self. This is in no way limited to sexuality but includes your relationships, your hobbies and interests, your style of dress, your friends, your home, your lifestyle and of course your career choices.

# 7. TIME TO RISE AND SHINE

'The potential benefits of physical activity to health are huge. If a medication existed which had a similar effect, it would be regarded as a 'wonder drug' or 'miracle cure'.'

Sir Liam Donaldson:
the former Chief Medical Officer of 2009

## What is The Rise Method™?

Rise; *an upward movement (noun), move from a lower position to a higher one; come or go up (verb)*

The Rise Method™ is our unique framework for a successful recovery from burnout. Over the years that I've been working in this role, I've tried and tested many different techniques, and I've now developed a framework that will help you recover from burnout if you follow the process. I chose the word 'rise' because of its positive connotations and because of the imagery the word creates. I think about changing from a stooped or crouched position metaphorically, to a tall and upright posture; there's also the imagery of the phoenix rising from the ashes and being reborn.

## Our philosophy (and the 'magic')

Helping a client successfully recover from burnout and then maintain good health comes through developing a relationship that extends into the many hours of the week that we're not with them, not just the time spent together. If the process is to be successful, then we will need to be able to influence the decisions you make throughout the process, and for a lot of that time, we won't be at your side. There are times when we will ask you to trust in the process, and give things a try. Being open-minded is crucial if you want to change. Asking yourself searching questions about your life load and lifestyle might require you to accept that aspects of your thinking up to now have not served you well. This might be hard to accept initially, but trust in the maxim that anyone can change their lives if they have a strong desire and belief that they can.

It is my belief that when an exceptional coach works with a client who has a strong desire to change, incredible things can happen. My own happiness and self-esteem are strongly underpinned by my consistent levels of fitness and healthy eating, and we will share with you the secret of how you can attain this same level of confidence about your health and wellbeing.

When a client comes to us, they are usually emotionally and physically exhausted, and very much in need of our help. In talking through the steps contained in The Rise Method™, we will demonstrate that if you follow and fully engage in the process, then you can and will recover your health. We'll ask questions to help you self-assess your position, and decide which package of services is best suited to your situation. These questions might include:

- Are you currently able to work?

- Have you been to see a doctor about how you're feeling?

- Have you been hospitalised for exhaustion, stress or other related conditions?

- Do you eat regular meals?

- Do you suffer from digestive problems?

- How many hours sleep do you typically get each night?

- How would you describe your stress levels?

- Do you struggle with your moods or find yourself behaving erratically or out of character?

- Do you feel there are not enough hours in the day for you to get everything done that is expected of you?

- Do you prioritise time for exercise and relaxation?

- Do you have back pain or suffer from headaches?

- Do you find that you get sick more often than usual, and take longer to recover?

- Do you struggle to get out of bed in the morning?

This is by no means a comprehensive list but it will help you to understand how you're feeling and where you need help.

## Principles of the Rise Method™

'Rise' is also an acronym; the 'R' stands for 'Review', the 'I' for 'Ignite', the 'S' for 'Strengthen' and the 'E' for 'Empower'. Each of these acronyms come together to represent The Rise Method™.

During the Review phase, we look at lifestyle factors as well as life load, and discuss your sleep patterns. We will also introduce you to your nutritional therapist who will go through your nutrition plans and goals, and perform some simple and non-invasive tests to measure stress and vitamin D3 levels. We also use a genetic test which enables us to establish what your requirements are for key vitamins such as vitamin D3, B6, B12 and other important aspects like anti-oxidants and cruciferous vegetable requirements, and carbohydrate, gluten and lactose sensitivity. Getting this part of the process right is very important for the overall success of the programme and making modifications to your diet usually results in some quick gains.

The Ignite phase is where we really get started with the exercise programme. The results of the genetic test are back and we can apply these to your nutrition plan. By this point you will be starting to notice the effects of your dietary changes, and starting to become more active.

During the Strengthen phase you will start to see changes in how you feel, both physically and mentally, and be proactively making some changes to your lifestyle. You will be exercising regularly, and implementing more of the suggested changes to your diet, resulting in further improvements in how you feel.

During the Empower phase you may be exercising independently as well as with us, and implementing more of the proposed lifestyle changes. We'll help you look to the future, and agree on what you will be doing to maintain your health and fitness and avoid slipping back into old habits. This step is about ensuring you have techniques and strategies to help prevent against burnout in the future, and to recognise the triggers and red flags that will inevitably appear again. It's very unlikely in life that you won't be faced with adversity or major challenges again, so you need to have a strategy to be able to manage. Remember, some of the aspects of your personality and temperament that might have made you more susceptible to burnout won't have completely disappeared. They will be very ingrained into your mind-set, so you'll need to be able to recognise when things are going awry, and be well-positioned to deal with whatever is being thrown at you whilst protecting your health.

## What we look at

### Life load questionnaire

The Rise Method™ places a lot of emphasis on life load. We define this as the daily load that you carry with you each day, every day. This includes family commitments; your job; your relationships (including spouse, partner, boss, staff); travel demands; the daily commute; your state of health (physical and mental); your financial commitments; your social life; your level of connectivity (mobiles, blackberry devices, pagers), and the stressors that are present in your life. It's really important for us to understand what your life load is, as we will have to work around this throughout the process. Sadly, just because you're burnt out, it doesn't mean that certain elements of your life load will disappear; we'll have to find a way of minimising their impact, or working with them. Understanding what those factors are in the crucial first step.

## Lifestyle review

This is different from the life load in that it focuses more on how you live your life and the choices you make. You'll be asked to outline what a typical day or week might look like for you, and how often you take time to relax, go on holiday or short breaks, or schedule some time for yourself. We'll explore patterns of behaviour, and identify areas where we need to focus.

## Adrenal Stress Index and Vitamin D3

We arrange for a saliva test to be taken that records your cortisol levels; high levels of cortisol are indicative of your overall levels of stress. In addition, high cortisol levels can affect your energy; cortisol inhibits the uptake of amino acids into the muscle cells, making it near impossible to fuel muscle cells when cortisol levels are too high for too long. It also inhibits bone formation and decreases calcium absorption in the intestine. So, when cortisol is high, there's no bone growth and no muscle growth. We measure your stress levels at the start of the process, and then again at the end to track the reduction.

We also do a vitamin D3 test to determine whether you have the right amounts in your body. Despite being a hormone not a vitamin, vitamin D3 is colloquially known as the 'sunshine vitamin' because we need direct sunlight in order to synthesise it. Because of the hemisphere in which we live here in Britain, it's common to find people are very low in D3, but boosting your intake is easy; if you are very deficient, you can either have an injection to get large amounts of it into you quickly, or powerful supplements can be prescribed and taken with food. If you are low but not dangerously so, then food should always be your primary source of vital nutrients.

## Nutritional therapy and genetic tests

We work with a team of very experienced nutritional therapists to undertake a complete review of what you eat and drink. This is a key part of the process and one area in which we can often make some quick gains. We will also do a genetic test with you, which I've found to be a real game-changer. It's a simple mouth swab, and the results help us understand how we can tailor an optimum nutrition plan which is very specific to you, rather than a generic plan or one based on educated guesswork.

## Tailored exercise sessions

Central to everything we do as part of the Rise Method™ is movement. We believe that exercise can be the most powerful mind-altering drug there is, and that a powerful combination of movement and empowerment can alter lives in a profound way. We'll design sessions according to what is appropriate; it might be a gentle walk in a park or peaceful setting or it might even be a walk around your back garden to start with, followed by some gentle stretching. It really depends on where we are starting out from. The team and I have worked with clients who have been unable to leave their home, but after we've worked together for a while we're meeting in the park, and their self-confidence is well on the way to being restored. Sometimes, a client is ready to start with something more dynamic, in which case we adapt as we go.

## Other disruptors

Sugar, alcohol, nicotine and caffeine are all examples of disruptors, and it's important that we understand what part these play in your lifestyle. It's common to find high levels of caffeine and alcohol (and therefore sugar) in the diet of someone who's burned out, and this can lead to poor absorption of nutrients. Add in a poor diet generally, and it's likely that your body is undernourished. If appropriate, blood tests can tell us if this is the case, and what restorative action we need to take.

Looking at alcohol intake can be a sensitive issue, but I personally have a lot of experience in this area, and I hope some of that can be useful to others. I understand that for some people, alcohol has been a prop and a comfort for them for many years, so we'll look at alcohol intake and patterns of drinking as part of a wider review of your lifestyle.

By focusing on disruptors, we will attempt to understand how we can substitute those things for healthier alternatives. Exercise is one such alternative. Typically, clients are drinking and smoking to try and relax their hyper-alert bodies and minds, and using sugar and caffeine to wake up and have the energy to get through the day. It's a see-saw motion of feeling exhausted so you pep yourself up with caffeine and sugar, then using alcohol and/or nicotine to wind down from a stressful day. Balancing that see-saw motion over time is a key focus.

## Sleep analysis

We'll ask you questions about your sleep patterns, to try and establish how much sleep you get and what the quality of sleep is like. Getting a good understanding of your sleep routine will be a priority. Usually our clients are sleep-starved and exhausted; we aim to give you the tools to improve your sleep routine, so that we can establish a base to build on. In our experience it's very hard to make changes when you are completely exhausted and sleeping very little, so this will be one of the first things we work on.

As Shakespeare said in my favourite of his plays, *Macbeth*:

> Sleep that knits up the ravell'd sleave of care,
> The death of each day's life, sore labour's bath,
> Balm of hurt minds, great nature's second course,
> Chief nourisher in life's feast…

Quite often burnout is driven by, or exacerbated by, a lack of sleep, as was the case with many of the executives I've mentioned in this book (Sam Smith and Antonio Horta Osorio, for example). Think back to Sam Smith's comment on how she could understand why sleep deprivation was and (in some parts of the world) still is used as a form of torture.

## Daily structure

Establishing a daily structure is really important throughout the recovery process. The structure might very simply be to ensure you've had a decent breakfast, had a walk and practised meditating for ten minutes each day. It doesn't have to be much, but it will help with the process. It is important to ensure that you don't take on too much either, and having a daily structure or routine gives that framework for the day. If you're still at work or planning to return, then understanding how you can structure your day so that you are able to manage your workload and stress levels is absolutely vital to continued good health. We will encourage you to map out your week, and ensure you have ring fenced times for light exercise; at least one opportunity to leave the office; rest breaks; adequate time to prepare for and travel to meetings to minimise stress, and marked in your diary when you are unavailable for meetings. (This could be marked in a diary as 'personal time', or simply as 'busy').

## Gratitude list

Successful recovery means finding meaning to your life, and not compromising on who you are. This includes learning to recognise and appreciate the things that really matter. Recovering from burnout requires you to recognise what you have and learn the value of it. Being loved, having a full and rich life, and being able to connect and empathise with others is hugely important. Find a vocation that allows you to do what you love. Many people I've spoken to whilst researching this book have changed their career paths after suffering from burnout. Very few have gone back to their old jobs, although some have, under new conditions. Something I've noticed people have found useful is a gratitude list. This is a simple list of things that you're grateful for. Some people aim to do this at the end of every day. It might be about your health, your pets, the weather, an act of kindness shown to you or done by you, or simply for feeling a little better than you did yesterday. I think everyone needs an occasional reminder of the good in their lives, and no more so than if you've suffered a burnout, when everything can seem very negative and overwhelming.

If you would like to know more about the Rise Method™ or you would like to register your interest, please visit www. leannespencer.co.uk or refer to the back of the book for other ways to contact me.

# 8. IS THERE A BETTER WAY?

So we've established that the current culture is now all about staying up-to-date, current and being 'on' all the time. Our working lives blur into our private lives, and we seem to have established a culture that rewards putting in endless hours and making sacrifices that come at the expense of family life and time to do other things like sport, exercise and other pastimes. Of course most of us need to work in order to feed and clothe ourselves and our families, but at an executive level, something else seems to be happening. We're losing more and more of our free time as our working hours overlap into personal time and we allow our gadgets to interrupt what time we do have to relax. The development of technology such as the mobile device and smart phone has gradually blurred the boundaries between work and leisure, and effectively ensured that whether we want to be or not, we're available 24/7, and never more than a swipe of our finger from news, social media, email, instant messaging, text messages and updates. Ask yourself whether you have a healthy set of rules around working practices, such as checking and responding to emails or taking calls outside of office hours, and I suspect most people would acknowledge there is an imbalance.

There are definitely other countries which appear to offer a better balance between work and home life than the UK, although it's also important to add there are many countries considerably worse than ours, in which to work. According to Organisation for Economic Cooperation and Development (OECD), the top ten happiest countries to live and work in are Australia, Iceland, Finland, Sweden, Norway, Switzerland, Canada, Austria, Netherlands and Denmark. I've selected just a few of these and analysed why they've earned that status.

## Norway

In Norway, the quality of living is very high, and this is in part due to the Norwegian culture relating to work, leisure and health. The Norwegians have a robust welfare system, which means there is a benefits system that protects those who need it, and supports parental leave, allowing families to achieve a better balance between their children and their careers. They enjoy many more public holidays than the UK, and employees are required to take five weeks annual leave. Vacations and free time are highly valued in Norway, and the working hours are typically 8am to 4pm, leaving time for other activities outside work. Most businesses are closed on Sundays too, which helps to create a culture where rest and relaxation is valued at least one day of the week – the pace of life is slowed right down. Even buses and trains run a reduced service on Sundays and there is no such thing as twenty-four hour shopping. All this allows people to prioritise family life and personal time.

Because of the vastness of the country, by default you will be more active in your daily life in Norway; exercise is almost essential, especially in winter months, and there is an abundance of clean, fresh air. Communities tend to cluster in much smaller groups, with lots of space both inside and outside the homes, and there are no overpopulated areas, which contribute to feelings of stress and pressure.

The Norwegian diet is rich in oils and fresh fish, and almost no fast food is available, so there are fewer issues around weight and other diet-related conditions (mental and physical). The scale and size of the country naturally decelerates the pace of life, which is probably why Norwegians experience less incidents of mental health in the workplace than we do.

## Sweden

At the time of writing, Sweden has begun trialling a six hour working day. Almost everyone has made the changes, from companies and corporations to retirement homes and hospitals. The hope and expectation is that it will result in improved productivity and a happier workforce, whilst also allowing people more time and energy for their personal lives. It's a bold move, but I'm willing to bet it pays off.

Interestingly, Toyota have been operating a reduced-hour policy for over thirteen years at their plant in Gothenburg. They report that it has resulted in increased profits, happier staff and a significantly lower turnover of staff. There are certain rules around the shorter day; for example, social media is banned, meetings are held only if absolutely required, and anything that might be distracting to workers is kept to a minimum.

Other corporate cultures are also waking up to the idea that it is possible to structure the working week in a more balanced way. At the time of writing, Uniqlo had just started offering its full-time Japanese workers the option of working a four-day week. There are no reports of them doing the same for the European or US workers yet though. On the face of it this appears to be a step in the right direction for work/life balance. Upon closer inspection, it's not quite as it appears to be. The four-day week will actually comprise ten-hour days rather than eight, and those who opt for it will have to work weekends and holidays. But having more options around working hours is a good start.

Similarly to Norway, the other benefits of Sweden include universal healthcare, five weeks annual leave and an incredible 480 days of parental leave on 80% pay. Notice that it is parental leave not maternity leave.

The air is clearer and more pure in Sweden, as is the water, and like Norway, the Swedes tend to live a very active lifestyle throughout the year.

It will be interesting to see if the six hour working day ever makes it to the UK, but there is much we could learn from the Swedes in terms of the work/life balance.

## Switzerland

Switzerland definitely has a much more relaxed working culture than most nations. Like the Scandinavian countries already mentioned, Switzerland offers a slower pace of life for its workers.

Shops and stores are closed on Sundays and generally it's a day for family and for leisure time, not commercialism. At Christmas, there is usually a complete shutdown from Christmas Eve to early January, which is effectively an extra week's vacation time in addition to the minimum of four week's annual leave. Taking holiday isn't something to feel guilty about, and longer breaks are encouraged.

The Swiss also value their lunch break; eating at your desk is uncommon and in some cases, frowned upon. I worked for a Swiss company, and we knew not to bother calling our Swiss colleagues between noon and 2pm because they would be in a restaurant eating lunch and we'd just get their voicemail.

According to OECD statistics, the Swiss earned approximately 40% more but worked on average 219 hours less than their US counterparts. Maternity leave is considerably better than the US or the UK; women receive fourteen weeks maternity leave at 80% of full pay, and they have a degree of flexibility about how many hours they wish to commit to when they return. For example, a woman might return to work but commit to 50% of her hours; she then has the option to work five half-days or two-and-a-half days per week. There's also more respect shown towards part-time workers in Switzerland; a part-time worker is paid a percentage of the salary a full-time worker would receive according to how many hours they do. If you lose your job, whether it's part-time or full-time, the Swiss government will give you 70-80% of your salary for up to eighteen months while you find a new job.

## Will the UK catch up?

Making some of these changes in the UK, though, is beyond the control of most of us; we are where we are. Governments and big business decides what our working conditions will be like at most if not all levels of the organisation. Some companies are starting to acknowledge and address the issue of mental health and burnout, however.

At least one of the big-four accountancy firms has a handful of senior partners who have nominated themselves to be 'Mental Health Champions'. The idea is that they are trained to be able to help people with mental health challenges, and are there to promote the idea that it's ok to talk about what's going for you in terms of stress, anxiety, depression or the pressure of work. The big aim is to try and catch burnout and mental health problems before they happen, and there are strict confidentiality agreements put in place (even with the senior partner's executive assistant), to encourage people to use the resource. Mental health charities and campaigners have welcomed the schemes, and generally it is hoped that by giving executives the channels to report how they're feeling, the stigma of mental health will start to become reduced.

Many of the people I spoke to whilst researching this book agreed that things were improving, there is still quite a way to go. Whilst our corporate cultures and working practices continue to challenge us, we need to take responsibility for our health as much as possible. We must commit to making good health our top priority.

To help you with this, I've created my top tips for a balanced lifestyle, which I hope will help you look at some of the aspects of your life where you can make positive changes.

**Ensure you get a good night's sleep.** Make this a priority and give thought to how you will ensure that you do get a restful night's sleep. Plan when you will put your mobile phone aside and start the process of unwinding; if you intend to get to bed by 10pm, start unwinding by 9pm by putting your phone onto silent or turning it off, and leaving it in another room or away from your bedside. You could do some gentle yoga stretches or go through a short meditative sequence or just sit quietly and spend a little time just boxing away your thoughts. Get a book (preferably a traditional paperback or hardback rather than a Kindle device) and read.

**Make sure you are hydrated all the time.** This is very easy to achieve as all it takes is small amounts of water, every thirty to sixty minutes, depending on what activity you're doing. If you are desk-based, having a tall glass full of water on your desk is good, but don't keep a larger glass or bottle by your desk as running out of water is an excellent opportunity to get up and take a short walk to the water cooler to refill your glass. This ensures you get up every hour and take a small amount of exercise. Your mind will thank you for this, and you are that little bit more active than you otherwise would have been.

**Regulate your caffeine and alcohol.** Both are classic examples of disruptors, and both taken in too high quantities will throw you out of balance. If you do drink caffeinated drinks, I recommend sticking to one or two cups per day maximum, and try and avoid caffeine after lunchtime. Similarly, alcohol disturbs all the processes in the body from digestion to sleep patterns, and it is a depressant. It will slow down the processes in the brain and the function of the central nervous system. If you're trying to achieve a balanced lifestyle, careful regulation of your alcohol intake is essential.

**Check your vitamin D3 levels.** Many of us are deficient in vitamin D3, although we might not know it. Common symptoms of a vitamin D3 deficiency include bone pain, muscle weakness, high blood pressure and depression. There are also links to dementia. Vitamin D3 is actually not a vitamin, but a steroid hormone that we are designed to obtain primarily through sun exposure rather than diet. In 2014, the National Institute for Clinical Excellence (NICE) estimated that around one in five adults and around one in six children may have low vitamin D3 status – that's an estimated ten million people across England. You can check your vitamin D3 levels as part of the Rise Method™ or by independently arranging a blood test.

**Eat regularly**. I've seen clients improve their mental health and alter their body composition by eating more. Eating small amounts regularly, providing it's the right type of food, can have a positive effect on how you feel. If you recall I mentioned earlier in this book that the brain has a very high glucose requirement; if you want to think clearly then you need to ensure your brain is getting enough fuel. Making sure you have the right balance of micronutrients (vitamins and minerals) is also essential for optimum health. For mental health, selenium, the B vitamins, vitamin D3, tryptophan, magnesium, calcium, and omega 3 and omega 6 are all important. The bottom line is that all the vitamins and minerals that our body is designed to work with are important, and so a balanced diet is crucial. If you are unsure whether you are eating a balanced diet, or would like to find out what your genetic requirements are, then get in touch with us.

**Practice mindfulness**. I've talked quite a bit about mindfulness in this book, but it can be a game changer. Few people I know or have come into contact with practice mindfulness and still have problems attaining balance in their lives. It won't remove your problems, stressors or life challenges, but it can provide you with a wonderful tool to help you manage these things, and it can be done anytime, anywhere and on your own.

**Exercise regularly**. Find something you enjoy, and if you are unsure what to do seek the help of an exercise professional. As I hope I've demonstrated in this book, exercise is a very powerful tool to help you manage stress, anxiety and depression, and to more generally ensure you stay fit and healthy in mind and body. I can't stress enough how important it is to keep moving, as our bodies were designed to do. The environment we live in now (especially our working environment), has been configured to ensure we move as little as possible. In fact there's now a term for it; obesogenic. This term refers to an environment that promotes weight gaining and one that is not conducive to weight loss. We need to move in order to thrive. Make it your priority to move as much as possible.

**Surround yourself with positive people**. I cannot stand to be around negative people. I've heard them described as 'mood hoovers' or 'energy vampires' and both expressions are very apt. We all have our low moments and I'm not for a minute suggesting that we abandon friends and colleagues who are having a hard time and need our support. We all can probably think of one or two people we know and spend time with that we might try and avoid because they are always moaning, being negative or talking about other people in a judgemental way. They are the people that will sap your energy. Surround yourself with positive people who prioritise their health and happiness, and enjoy the positive benefits this will have on you. Encourage each other to be your best selves.

**Remove monkey-brain distractions from your life**. Monkey-mind is a Buddhist expression which refers to the incessant chatter that goes on in our heads. It is estimated that the mind produces up to 100,000 thoughts a day, which seems like an astonishing amount of thinking. We are also bombarded with messages through advertising, mobile devices, email etc. If we want to be able to filter out the junk from the important stuff, we need to minimise the monkey brain activity. It was suggested to me a few months ago, on a programme I'm doing, that I avoid all the news (print and online), remove myself from social media and focus only on what's going to make me successful. Streamlining the amount of messages you allow in (I accept some will be subconscious), and controlling the amount of content you put in front of yourself will enable you to think with more clarity and purpose. If you give it thought, there are very few 'urgent' news articles that you really need to know about. Most of it is propaganda to some extent, or things that you can live without knowing all about. Most of it is also drama; who's wearing what, who's sleeping with who or who's let themselves go. Try going without it for a few weeks and see if you feel bereft – I suspect you won't.

**Make sure everything you do is an honest reflection of your authentic self.** This is the most important tip of all. If you can crack this, then you'll find everything else much simpler. Everyone I've interviewed for this book, spoken to as a friend or colleague or have worked with as a client, has got to where they're at with their health because in some area of their life they were not being authentic to themselves. Think back to the example I gave about Vicky Beeching; she found herself having to deal with a very serious auto-immune condition because she was suppressing her sexuality. Other executives I mentioned in this book have ended up abruptly leaving their jobs because they don't reflect their values, principles or beliefs. Search within yourself to make sure what you do and what you stand for is reflected in the choices you've made in your life; that includes your job, your partner, where you live, the clubs and associations you represent. Look hard and then have the courage to make the changes that are necessary to fulfil that authentic self. That's the key to good health and happiness, and it's there within you if you look for it.

# APPENDIX A: I BELIEVE...

I believe in the potential to radically improve human lives when diet and exercise combine with a strong desire to change.

I believe that anyone can change their lives if they have a strong desire and belief that they can.

I believe that when an exceptional coach works with a client who has a strong desire to change, incredible things can happen.

I believe that exercise can be the most powerful mind-altering drug there is.

I believe that a powerful combination of movement and empowerment can alter lives in a profound way.

I believe there is an astonishing power at the intersection of determination and desire.

I believe that everyone has the ability to change direction. Nothing is impossible.

I believe too many people suffer from low self-esteem. This is a travesty and cripples personal development and personal happiness.

I believe in the wonders of the human body and what it will do for you if you treat it with respect.

I believe in the power of two people focused on a common goal with an unswerving desire to make it happen.

I believe that every client we work with should be treated with empathy, congruence and unconditional positive regard.

I believe everything we do for our clients should represent our core values of **integrity, loyalty, focus** and **success**.

I believe in what I do. It works.

# APPENDIX B:
# I DO WHAT I DO BECAUSE....

I like to help people.

I believe exercise has a profound effect on mental as well as physical health.

I believe my own happiness and self-esteem are strongly underpinned by my fitness and healthy eating.

Helping people manage life-threatening and health-threatening conditions such as stress, anxiety and depression is very important to me as the cost of these conditions to the sufferer, their friends and family and the economy as a whole is vast and underappreciated.

I want to build a business based on what I love doing and wholeheartedly believe in.

I love to encourage both men and women (but especially women) to be proud of their appearance and to feel confident about exercise.

I love seeing my clients grow in confidence, expand their horizons, attract new opportunities and achieve their goals.

Our bodies are meant to move so I spend my time showing clients how to do this safely and enjoyably in order to prolong their health span.

Positive mental health is critical. Exercise and diet are the cornerstones of good health, and I strive to help my clients recognise that and learn to make those things part of their daily lifestyle.

Seeing a client develop and open up in front of our eyes as a result of our programmes is a wonderful feeling.

Running this business allows me to stay active and talk about topics that I'm passionate about.

# RECOMMENDED READING

### Burnout, Lifestyle and Meditation

*Thrive* by Arianna Huffington

*Fried* by Joan Borysenko

*Mindfulness* by Gill Hasson

*The Chimp Paradox* by Professor Steve Peters

### Diet and Nutrition

*Serve to Win* by Novak Djokovic

*Eat Your Heart Out* by Felicity Lawrence

*Not on the Label* by Felicity Lawrence

*Optimum Nutrition for the Mind* by Patrick Holford

### Inspiration

*Entrepreneur Revolution* by Daniel Priestley

*Bold as Brass* by Hillary Devey

*The Virgin Way* by Sir Richard Branson

*Life and Limb* by Jamie Andrew

### City Culture

*A Colossal Failure of Common Sense* by Larry McDonald

*Leaders Eat Last* by Simon Sinek

*Cityboy* by Geraint Anderson

*Liars Poker* by Michael Lewis

# ACKNOWLEDGMENTS

It's an incredible feeling to have planned, written and published a book, but there are many people that helped me along the way.

I'd like to thank three people for helping and encouraging me to write this book now, not later or next year, or whenever I've got more time. The first person is Daniel Priestley, for writing the inspirational book *Entrepreneur Revolution*, which resulted in me signing up to the KPI programme. This book would not exist if it wasn't for Daniel, so thank you. The other two people to whom I owe thanks are Lucy McCarraher and Joe Gregory for their words of wisdom and guiding me through the publishing process.

Huge thanks to my contributors Sarah R, Ker Tyler and Rachel S, who generously shared their personal stories in the book and made it much richer as a result. I am very grateful to you all.

A big thank you to my mum Carolyn Walsham for her eagle-eyed proof-reading, and to Antonia, my partner, who may or may not have minded me spending so much time in my study writing, but was considerate enough to pretend she didn't.

Finally, a heartfelt thank you to you, my readers. I sincerely hope this book has been useful to you, and that it helps, even in a small way.

# THE AUTHOR

Leanne Spencer began her career in sales, marketing and account management, and spent over fifteen years working for a handful of start-ups and large corporates before leaving to set up her own business doing something that she felt was more meaningful and authentic. In 2012, after suffering from burnout, 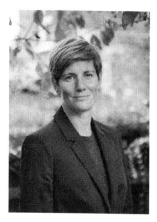 she left the City and set about establishing herself as a fitness entrepreneur, author, blogger and health coach.

Leanne is the founder of the personal training and well-being company Bodyshot Performance Limited, which specialises in bringing the science of genetics to women's fitness, and is fast becoming a leading authority on how to use exercise and lifestyle interventions to help executives recover from burnout.

*Rise and Shine* is Leanne's first book, but she regularly blogs for a leading business accelerator website, and frequently contributes to articles in health and fitness magazines. Leanne has her own blog, which she regularly updates with insightful and relevant content, and is active on social media. She lives in South London with her partner and two cats, but escapes to the countryside whenever possible.

You can follow Leanne on Twitter using the handle @riseshinemethod, sign up to her blog at https://bodyshotblog. wordpress.com/ or visit the website at www.leannespencer. co.uk.

Printed in Great Britain
by Amazon